spice spa

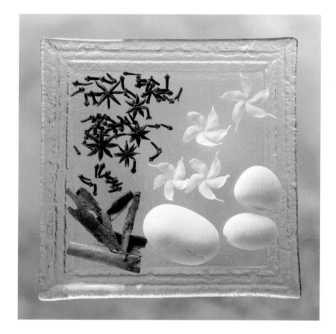

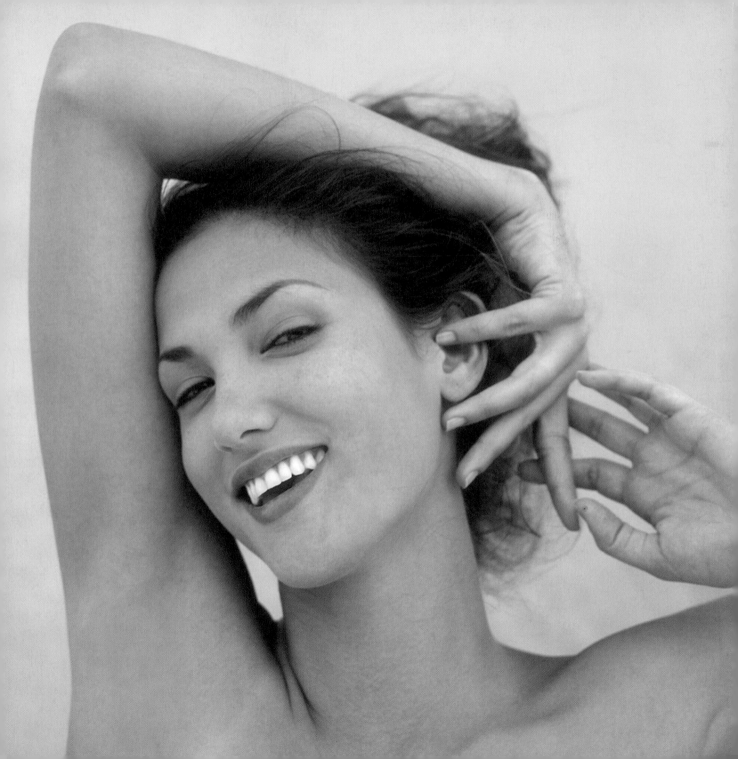

spice spa

**Rubs, scrubs, masks, and baths
for re-claiming health, beauty,
and internal balance**

Susannah Marriott

CARROLL & BROWN PUBLISHERS LIMITED

To baby Berry, who grew as I wrote.

This edition published in 2003 by
Carroll & Brown Publishers Limited
20 Lonsdale Road
London NW6 6RD

Project Editor Anna Amari-Parker
Managing Art Editor Jacqueline Duncan
Photographer Jules Selmes

A CIP catalogue record for this book is available
from the British Library

ISBN 1-903258-58-8

10 9 8 7 6 5 4 3 2 1

Reproduced by Emirates Printing Press (L.L.C.),
United Arab Emirates
Printed for Imago in Singapore

Disclaimer: This book is not a therapeutic or a weight loss
resource. If you have a skin condition, high blood
pressure, or are pregnant, seek medical advice before
doing any of these practices. The author and publishers
disclaim any liability from any injury occurring in the
practice of the treatments outlined in the book.

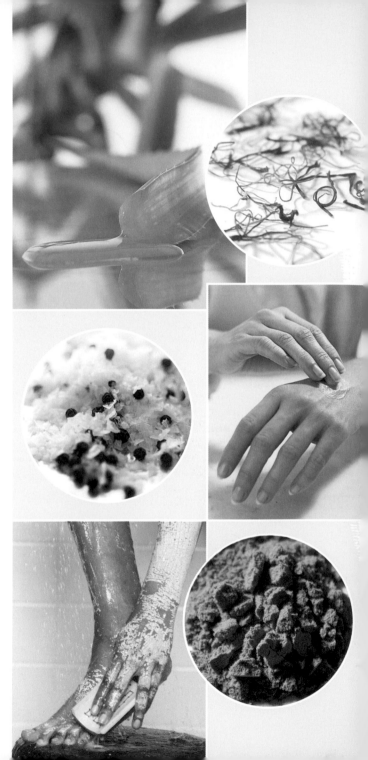

Contents

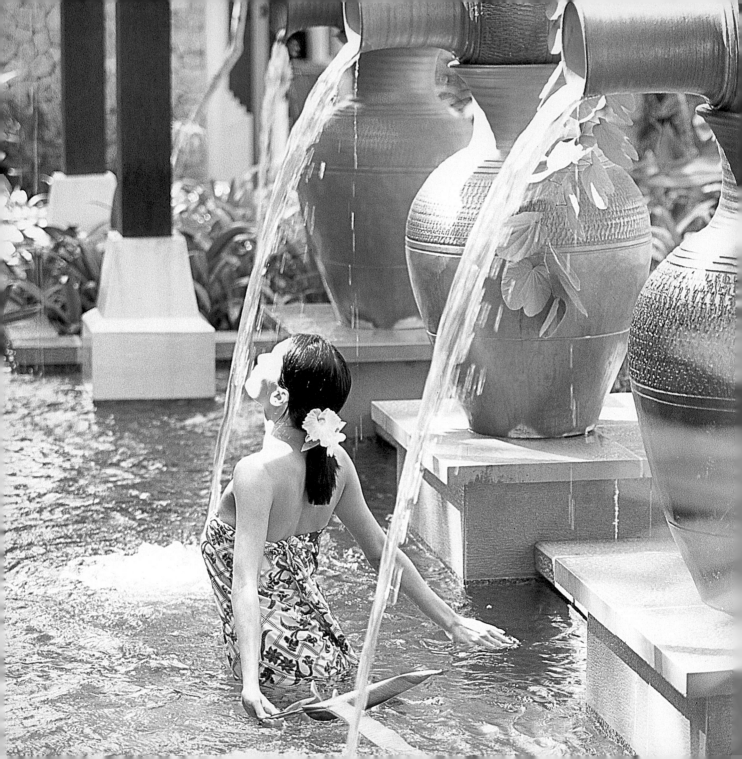

Introduction

For centuries, the scents of the spice rack have conjured up in the West the exotic sounds, sights, and smells of the East: the burning of incense in temples, the saffron-colored robes of holy men, the gloss of henna-tinted locks. Today, spices are being "rediscovered" and have increasingly come to occupy pride of place in massage, bathing rituals, and other body-pampering techniques at luxury spas throughout Asia from Bangkok to Bali. Top-notch spas in the West have also recognized this trend and are keen to emulate Eastern holistic mind-body relaxation techniques and beauty treatments blended from indigenous spices, herbs, and local healing plants. These almost mystical recipes are now being transported from the peaceful foothills of the Himalayas and the coast of Kerala to the bustling cities of the West, where an increasingly overworked population has welcomed all-natural, holistic beauty treatments with open arms. The relaxation and meditation traditions of Asian cultures have become the most recent, must-have beauty treatments for stressed urbanites in search of total mind-body-spirit rejuvenation. In this book, I have adapted some of the most luxurious spa treatments on offer at the world's exclusive beauty centers. There are over 100 easy-to-follow recipes and beauty rituals (based on organic spices, herbs, tropical fruits, nut oils, seaweed, and mud) that you can create in your own bathroom. Choose from facial cleansing powders, steams, and masks; exfoliating body polishes, wraps, and massage oils; sensual bath milks and softening foot soaks; or deep-conditioning hair creams and nourishing natural colorants. I hope these recipes result in not just silken skin and a beautifully toned body, but the heightened peace of mind and energy levels that are universally recognized signs of beauty.

Susannah Marriott

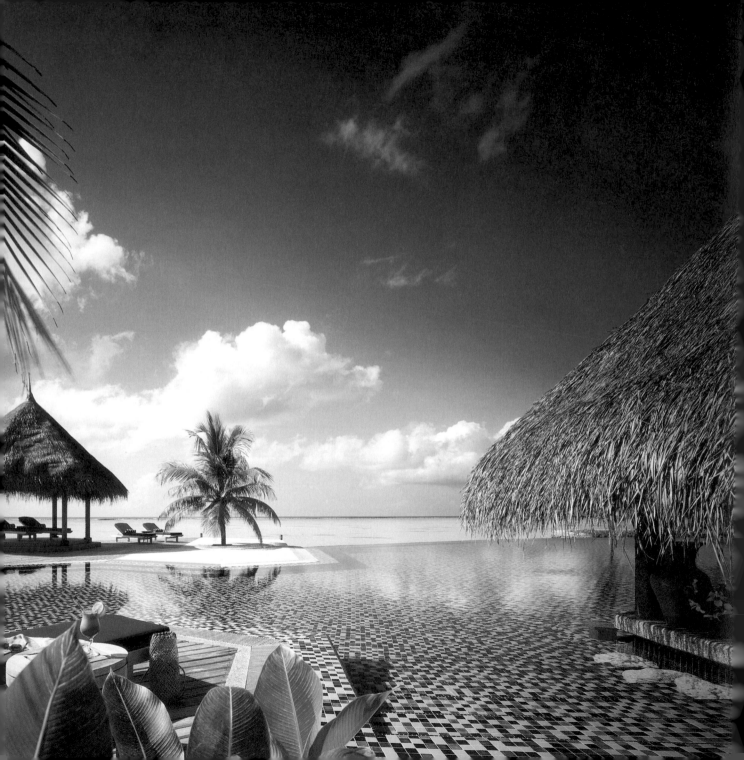

The luxury of spices

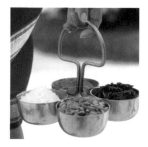 Most spices are native to Asia and archaeological finds reveal that they have been traded as precious commodities since the earliest recorded times. Then, as now, they were used to beautify and perfume the body and the home, as well as cure ills and flavor food. Traditional health and beauty secrets from India, Indonesia, China, and Japan—where spicy oils and scrubs are combined with massage and water-based therapies—have now passed into mainstream Western beauty care via the route of luxury health spas and holistic retreats. These treatments are prized for rebalancing the mind and smoothing, relaxing, and reviving the body.

Precious spices

Historically considered to be worth their weight in gold, aromatic sensual delights such as black pepper, cinnamon, saffron, and vanilla can transform the taste and nutritional properties of humble foodstuffs into a feast fit for gods, enhance the atmosphere in a room, and cure illness either through ingestion or a topical application to the skin. Countless wars have been waged and entire continents colonized in the pursuit of these wondrous natural products.

The power of spices

Spices have managed to maintain an aura of sensual exotic luxury, an edge that other tropical imports such as sugar, tea, coffee, and chocolate—equally miraculous at the time of their discovery in the Old World—have now lost. Spices still conjure up images of indulgence and plenty, of abundance and exotic allure. They evoke the signature flavors and scents of diverse cultures, whether in spicy combinations such as Indian *masala* powder, or blended into hair conditioners, body scrubs, Ayurvedic skincare treatments, and Middle Eastern bathing rituals.

These aromatic substances signified wealth, power, and influence, and came to define much of early economic and cultural contact between East and West. From the 3rd century BCE, the Silk Road, extending from China through central Asian trading posts to the cities of Persia, Syria, Greece, and the Roman Empire, saw spices being exchanged for other, equally precious, cargo. Anise, ginger, cassia, and rose trees left China in return for Roman glass and gold; from India came sandalwood and pepper; Persia brought peaches, pears, pistachio nuts, frankincense, and myrrh.

Each time they exchanged hands, the price of spices soared and these luxuries became very costly and sought-after. Western traders determined to access a direct route; Roman sailors discovered they could sail from Egypt's Red Sea coast to India and back within a year using the strength of monsoon winds. In the 15th century, the search for that fabled source of spices—the Indies—led Europeans to discover new sea routes, and triggered centuries of global exploration and exploitation.

By the 17th century, English, French, and Dutch traders were competing with the Portuguese for the massive, fail-safe profits from indigenous spices by setting up colonies and trading ventures in a frenzy to reap the riches that the spice lands and routes had to offer. The Dutch East India Company, founded on the trade of cloves, became the world's richest company, trading spices for salt in the Persian Gulf; salt for cloves in Zanzibar; cloves for gold in India; gold for Chinese tea and silk; Japanese copper for silk; and copper for spices in the East Indies.

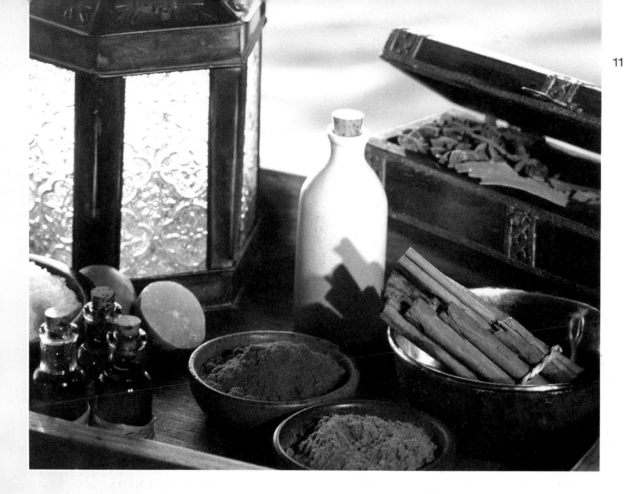

Healing essences

What was the driving force behind such demand? Spices were perceived as substances that could cure body and mind, and as ingredients in products able to rebalance the body and elevate the spirit. Alongside the spice trade *per se*, the spice secrets of medicine and preventative healthcare passed between European traders and Asian herbal healers.

Neolithic spice-grinding stones discovered in Pakistan, and equipment for the distillation of essential oils dating from 3000 BCE, uncovered at the foothills of the Himalayas, show just how long humankind has cultivated an understanding of the health-giving qualities of spices. Cinnamon was imported for use in Egyptian massage oils from around 1450 BCE, while the *Ebers* papyrus (*c.* 1500 BCE)—the foundation of Greek, Roman, and Arabic healthcare—listed the medicinal use of 700 herbs and spices in ancient Egypt such as saffron, sesame, cardamom, and cassia.

Beauty secrets of the ancients

The ancient Greeks favored using imported spices such as cassia, black pepper, and ginger, alongside native coriander, saffron, and poppy seeds in their healing practices. Adopting much herbal lore from ancient Egypt, they combined spices with massage and water-based treatments, stirring mustard powder, for instance, into warm baths to soothe aching limbs and boost circulation. The first Western herbal, *De Materia Medica*, written by the Greek physician Dioscorides (40-90 CE), set out the use of around 600 medicinal plants and was still consulted by the 17th century.

During the Roman Empire, spices formed a key healing tool. Spicy tisanes, decoctions, pastes, and powders were recommended to ease common ailments and serious diseases in conjunction with massage and water treatments. The Romans espoused the life-enhancing qualities of water and built public baths, where spice-oil massages were on offer; spices were also burned and scattered to perfume private homes as well as public places.

After the fall of Rome in 476 CE, Baghdad became the epicenter for riches and knowledge from the East, as well as the hub of the spice trade within a thriving Islamic empire extending from Spain into central Asia. Physicians, herbalists, and traders benefited from the rich exchange of herb and spice lore that combined Indian and Chinese healthcare systems with Greek and Roman medical knowledge. The physician Ibn Sina (980-1037 CE) charted the healing use of spices and perfected the process of distilling essential oils from plants. Once the texts of Islamic medicine (or *Unani Tibb*), which drew on Greek and Roman wisdom, were translated into Latin, they transmitted this medical know-how.

Spiritual spices

Arab traders, keen to conceal the origins of valuable spices in order to maintain their monopoly on trade, attributed supernatural properties to these plants. This helps to explain the enduring mystique surrounding spices: perhaps because of their incredible health-giving properties, they have been

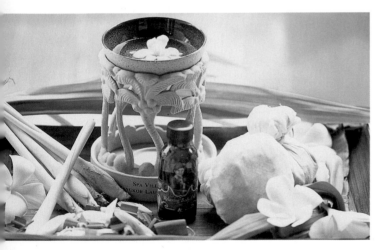

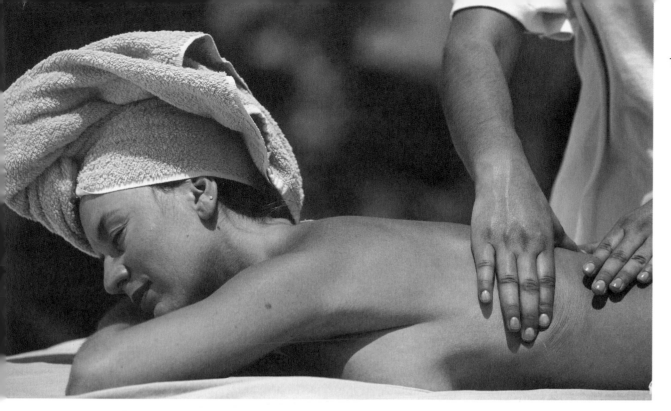

considered to be magical and God-given across cultures, instant conduits to the spiritual realm.

From time immemorial, ceremony and devotion have been intertwined with the cultivation and use of spices. In ancient India and Mesopotamia, they were burned as incense to connect the earth and the heavens through a spiral of smoke.

The healing properties of spices and their blending with oil for massage were also described in the Hindu *Vedas* (*c.* 1500 BCE), the world's earliest written prayers and religious rites. The Bible, too, records the use of several spice-containing anointing recipes evocative of ancient Egyptian incense mixtures.

Sandalwood, cloves, and a variety of other spices are still in use within the Buddhist communities of southeast Asia and the Hindu culture of India to promote meditation, relaxation, and deepen spirituality. Modern-day spice beauty treatments choose to draw on the power of these aromatic substances to engage the spirit and open the mind. They offer the ultimate luxury—time for yourself to tune out of daily stresses and spiritually reconnect with your spirit and the natural world.

India's spice tradition

Many Westerners have been introduced to Ayurveda—India's 5,000-year-old healthcare tradition—through its spice-enhanced beauty treatments: massages, body oils, purifying wraps, masks, and scrubs. Each spice and herb (over 2,000 are used in poultices, pastes, oils, juices, and teas) is recognized for its unique therapeutic properties and corresponds to one of five elements (ether, air, fire, water, or earth) and one of six tastes (sweet, sour, salty, pungent, bitter, or astringent). Every spice and herb has either a heating or cooling effect on the body that helps to bring it back to its natural equilibrium. Different Ayurvedic combinations of spices are specifically suited to each of the three doshas (*see box*).

Ayurvedic massage

Massage is a key Ayurvedic healing technique, a way of ensuring that life energy, or *prana*, flows freely through the body's channels clearing up blockages that lead to ill health and unhappiness. Indian massage, like yoga, works on the 107 *marma* points (energy junctions) and the seven chakras (energy centers) that run down the body. Carefully blending herb and spice oils brings the doshas back into balance and leaves skin glowing.

The seasons & your skin

As the doshas of the seasons flow into one another, your skin's needs change. Adapt your beauty care regime to echo this seasonal movement.

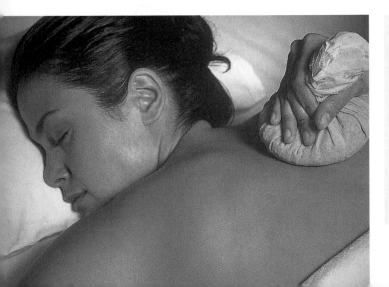

What are doshas?
Everything in the universe is composed of five elements. These create three essential energies—or doshas—when combined: vata (air and ether); pitta (fire and water); kapha (earth and water). You are born with a unique combination of these three types. Identifying which one predominantly governs your constitution will enable you detect any imbalances in your body and make changes before they lead to illness or disrupt wellbeing.

Assessing your dosha

Each one of us has a predominance of one or, more often, two types of dosha. The chart below will help you identify which description most closely resembles you.

	Vata	Pitta	Kapha
Body shape	slight	medium build	heavy build
Face shape	angular	heart-shaped	round
Skin type	thin, dry	reddish	oily, thick
Perspiration	light	profuse	moderate
Appetite	variable	dominant	steady
Speech	rapid	penetrating	monotonous
Movement	quick	dynamic	slow
Energy	nervous	motivated	enduring
Enthusiasm	volatile	passionate	grounded
Mindset	changeable	sharp	relaxed
Mode of action	erratic	confident	methodical
Key emotional trait	excitability	fieriness	tenderness
Sleep pattern	light	sound	deep
Stress response	flight	fight	freeze

Spring: As winter turns into spring, the energy of pitta predominates. This is a good time to detox after the stagnation of winter. Use a sandalwood face mask as you relax in the bath. Choose products with detoxifying fennel and black pepper.

Summer: Counterbalance the fire element of this hot and dry pitta season with coconut or sunflower oil body massages each morning before a cool shower. Rub your scalp and the soles of the feet with coconut oil before going to bed. To promote sleep, put 2-3 drops of sandalwood essential oil on your pillow. Choose cooling products with sandalwood, coriander, and lemon grass.

Fall: Vata gains the ascendancy with cold, windy, and drying influences. Fight the appearance of wrinkles with sesame oil body massages before a warm morning shower. Choose products with moisturizing and emollient avocado and almond.

Winter: In midwinter and early spring, kapha rules with a cold, damp heaviness that makes skin sluggish and dull-looking. Use warming oil treatments and take hot showers, saunas, and steam baths. Choose products with warming nutmeg, ginger, and black pepper.

The Chinese Tao of beauty

In China, beauty care techniques are inseparable from healthcare remedies. A healthy body equals a balanced mind and vice versa because the eternal flow of universal chi energy moves through and all around you.

Herbal healing using plants and spices is pivotal to Chinese healthcare. Over 5,700 plants are used in Traditional Chinese Medicine (TCM). Some ancient 4,000-year-old manuscripts, such as *The Yellow Emperor's Classic of Internal Medicine* (*c.* 200 BCE-100 CE), detail herbal healing recipes still prescribed today! China's earliest medical textbooks also describe the yin or yang properties of herbs and spices (*see right*); their warming or cooling effects on the body; their corresponding tastes (sour, bitter, sweet, pungent, or salty), and the reactions these have on related organs and body systems. Included are accounts of herb and spice-infused oil massages, which were such an integral part of TCM that the Imperial Court itself would sponsor massage departments within its medical establishments.

Yin & yang

Chi, or life's energy, runs effortlessly into and through a healthy, balanced body, generating glowing skin, glossy hair, and overall vitality. TCM teaches that two interdependent forces—yin and yang—govern everything in nature, including the human body. Yang is hot, dominant, positive, light, masculine, and active. It symbolizes the day, upward movement, and the exterior. Yin is cool, calm, dark, feminine, and passive. It represents the night, downward movement, and the interior. Each is constantly turning into and defining the other. TCM recognizes that we are comprised of the same elements that make up the universe—wood, fire, earth, metal, and water—so different body parts and emotions, like the seasons, are governed by one of these five energies (*see opposite*). When these forces are in equilibrium, wellbeing ensues, and TCM offers practical ways to adapt the body to inevitable fluctuations.

Chi energy routes

According to Chinese medicine, 12 energy pathways, or meridians, run through the body carrying chi to all the vital organs. Ill health, stress,

---

Yin and yang foods and spices

Heating yang foods: Most spices, including cinnamon, ginger, and nutmeg.

Cooling yin foods: Banana, coconut, watermelon, and seaweed.

Neutral foods (neither yin nor yang): Rice, black sesame seeds, Korean white ginseng, papaya, and soya beans.

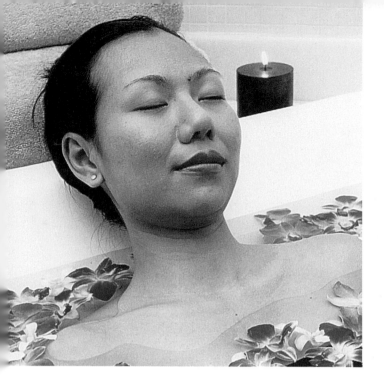

The five elements

Wood: Spring; windy; sour; astringent; liver, gall bladder, eyes, tendons.

Fire: Summer; hot; bitter; cooling; heart, small intestine, tongue, blood vessels.

Earth: Late summer; damp; sweet; tonic; spleen, stomach, mouth, flesh.

Metal: Fall; dry; pungent; stimulant; lungs, large intestine, nose, skin.

Water: Winter; cold; salty; fluid-draining; kidneys, bladder, bones, ears, hair.

or an unhealthy lifestyle cause blockages within these channels. Acupuncture, acupressure, and chi gong movements (a Chinese exercise system) stimulate a total of 365 key acupoints along these pathways to clear energy disruptions and free up the flow of chi.

A spice for every season

Eat in accordance with the season at hand to fight climatic excesses and restore the body's disrupted balance. This manifests as cold, dry, damp, wind, heat, or fire-related symptoms. Take cooling yin foods to counter physical heat or "hot" inflamed conditions such as sore throats and skin flare-ups. In cool weather, or when signs of "cold" conditions start to show—pallid skin or chilled feet—restore balance by eating warming yang foods. Ginger, cinnamon, and ginseng are considered to be "upper"

or "ruler herbs," valued for their capacity to boost the flow of chi and blood around the body and increase longevity and wellbeing.

Re-energizing and detoxifying

The beneficial effects of detoxification really show up on your skin, the body's largest organ. Coconuts, bananas, sesame oil and seeds, soya sauce, and rice—all used in Chinese detox regimes—richly nourish skin. Other skin-saving superfoods include cherries, melon, avocado, watercress, walnuts, and high-collagen treats such as honey and safflower oil. TCM also recommends cleansing herbal teas to revitalize the body from within. Ginseng tea is an effective body booster, and clove tea makes a good digestive tonic.

Asian health & beauty

Southeast Asian countries like Indonesia, Thailand, and Japan are a veritable treasure trove of ancient health and beauty traditions, which find expression through all-natural recipes and massage techniques.

Indonesia

There is a little-known yet long established holistic healing tradition in Indonesia, known as *Jamu*, in which beauty care is combined with preventative medicine. Using the leaves, roots, and bark of more than 1,000 indigenous plants, *Jamu* healers create teas, tisanes, decoctions, infusions, powders, pastes, massage oils, lotions, cosmetics, and pills to heal, rebalance, and beautify. *Jamu* is used to treat every ill from the common cold to high blood pressure, cholesterol levels to rheumatism, but it is perhaps becoming best recognized for its role in beautifying. A growing number of holistic spas in Bali, Java, and other Indonesian islands are adapting this rich heritage and applying it to treatments for clear skin, glossy hair, a firm bust, and fat reduction. The best-

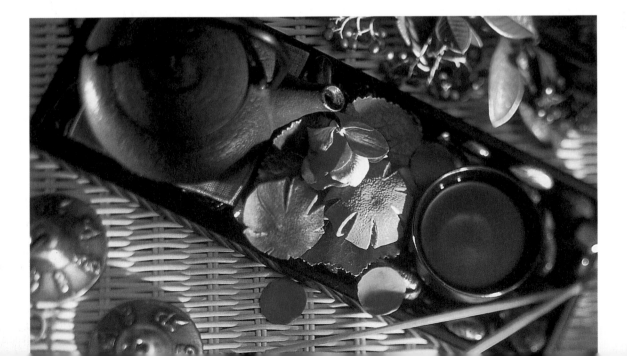

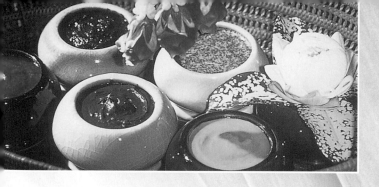

preserved branch of *Jamu* stems from the women's quarters at the royal palaces of Java, where beautifying techniques, including floral baths, incense-infused steam treatments, and spicy paste massages were administered to exfoliate and soften the skin.

Indonesian massage, known as *pijat* or *urut*, combines various pressure-point and energy-raising techniques with smooth strokes and curative oils made from both native and imported spices, including coconut, ginger, and turmeric. This type of massage promotes good health through relaxation and rebalancing, but it is also used to heal more serious ailments like fractured bones.

Thailand

Traditional Thai healing is threefold. Firstly, plant recipes are prescribed to bring body and mind into equilibrium. Secondly, meditation and spirituality are encouraged to rebalance every part of the system. Thirdly and, best known of all, is *nuad bo'rarm*, the traditional Thai massage technique that fuses strokes and acupressure point stimulation with flowing movements that manipulate the body into yoga postures. Thai massage prevents ill health and helps to cure ailments by promoting the flow of energy along 10 key energy lines (or *sen*) in the body. Thai masseurs give your body a beneficial workout by pressing and stretching skin and muscles using hands, feet, elbows, and thumbs. Rejuvenated and glowing skin alongside postural improvement are the most noticeable benefits.

Japan

The Japanese beauty ideal places a heavy emphasis on purification (both spiritual and physical) through bathing and the use of herbal formulas containing native plants and fruit. Traditional Japanese herbal medicine, or *kampoh*, originated around the 5th century CE with the arrival of Korean physicians and Buddhist monks, who brought to Japan the healing practices of China. *Kampoh* formulas are very measured and use between five and 10 ingredients. Unlike the raw contents of Chinese herbalism, many of these are freeze-dried.

The Japanese are also expected to bathe daily, either at home, in a communal bathhouse (*sento*), or an outdoor spring (*onsen*) following Shinto rituals.

In keeping with Chinese healthcare concepts, the Japanese have always highly prized the art of massage. *Anma*, the oldest and most indigenous form of Japanese massage, relaxes and restores the whole body, whereas with shiatsu, the Japanese healing art of touch, localized pressure is applied to key acupoints and meridians using the fingertips, thumbs, elbows, knees, and feet.

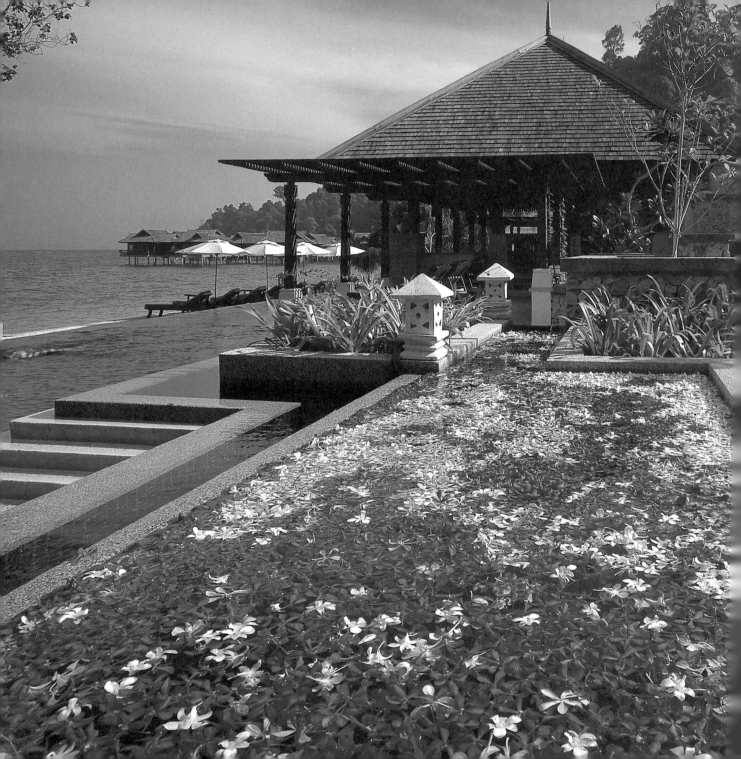

2

Spa treatments from around the world

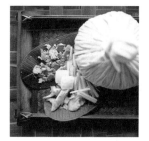

Throughout the centuries and around the world, from the Buddhist temples of Thailand to the tribal homesteads of India, from the palaces of Indonesia to sultry Arab deserts, from the islands of the Caribbean to the dressing tables of Western Europe, spices have been ground, chopped, blended, and infused. Applied to the face and the body, they promise a clear complexion with toned and revitalized skin, and beautifully conditioned hair. And for a total mind, body, and spirit experience, these scents help the spirit soar.

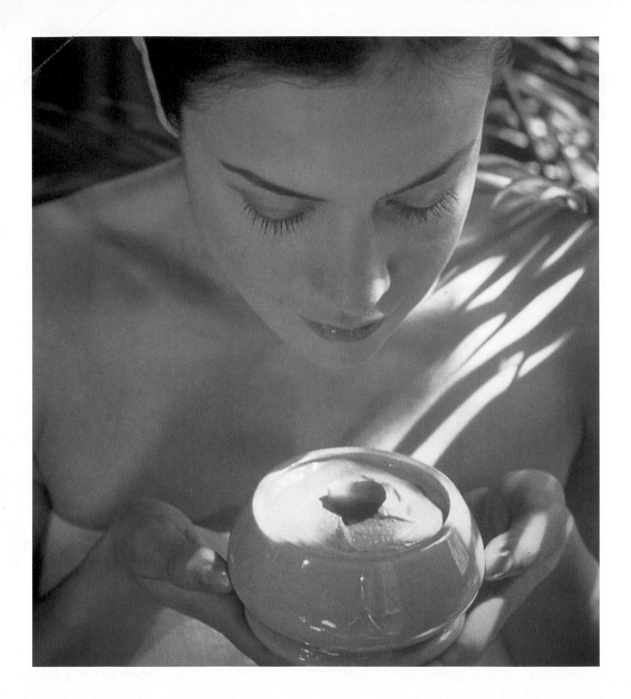

spice blends for the face

In the Ayurvedic tradition, blends of spices and other kitchen staples with sacred associations (like honey, milk, rice) are applied to the face to rebalance the energies within the body. When combined with massage strokes to stimulate vital energy areas, such concoctions are said to bring to the recipient the benefits of a natural face-lift. Observe how your skin changes with the seasons and learn to echo this ever-moving natural cycle by creating and adapting spice-filled products for your face. In winter, you might need more nurturing emollients to retain moisture and warmth, whereas in summer, lighter masks and cooling toners might feel more appropriate. Live in balance with the natural world by listening to your skin's beauty care needs as it effortlessly tunes into its environment.

Cleansing powders & pastes

Ayurvedic practitioners advocate limiting the use of soap to cleanse skin except for sandalwood, which should be used sparingly. Instead, they recommend a balanced mixture of facial cleansing powders and pastes, specifically suited to your individual constitution or dosha type (*see pages 14-15*). Depending on your given dosha, Ayurveda even prescribes the optimum water temperature at which to splash your skin after cleansing. For an intense body cleansing experience, try the Total Detoxification ritual (*see pages 52-53*), which aims to purify the body in spring and fall in harmony with the changing of the seasons.

Vatas

- 2-5 drops sesame or avocado oil
- 1 tsp ground almonds
- ½ tsp powdered milk
- 1 tbsp milk

Gently wipe away any make-up and the day's impurities with a few drops of sesame or avocado oil on a cotton ball. Moisten the almonds and powdered milk with a little milk. Gently rub over your face and neck. Splash off with hot water.

Pittas

- 2-5 drops sunflower or coconut oil
- 1 tsp ground almonds
- ½ tsp ground coriander seeds
- ½ tsp powdered milk
- 1 tbsp cream

Gently wipe away any make-up and the day's impurities with some drops of sunflower or coconut oil on a cotton ball. Moisten the almonds, coriander, and milk with the cream. Smooth onto your face and neck. Rinse with cool water.

Kaphas

- 2-5 drops sweet almond oil
- 1 tsp ground oatmeal
- ½ tsp powdered milk
- 1 tsp grated lemon peel
- 1-2 tbsp orange blossom water

Gently wipe away any make-up and the day's impurities with a few drops of sweet almond oil on a cotton ball. Moisten the oatmeal, powdered milk, and lemon peel with a little orange blossom water. Apply to face and neck. Splash off with warm water.

Facial steaming

For deeper cleansing once a week, harness the power of water vapor to draw out toxins, unblock clogged pores, and plump up tired, lifeless skin. For dry or mature complexions, let the steam penetrate your skin for five minutes. For normal or oily skin, extend exposure for up to 10 minutes. Pat dry with a soft, clean towel and add moisturizer while your face is still warm and damp (*see pages 32-33*). These treatments are especially effective for revitalizing dull winter skin.

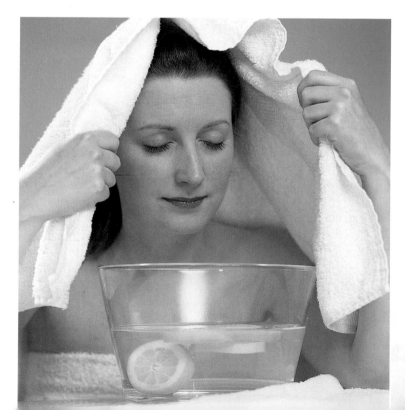

Normal skin

To a basin of boiling water, add 2 drops of essential oil of lemon grass and 2 drops of essential oil of mandarin. Cover your head with a towel, close your eyes, and relax into the steam for 10 minutes.

Oily skin

To a basin of boiling water, add 3 drops of essential oil of ginger and 4 slices of lemon. Cover your head with a towel, close your eyes, and relax into the steam for 10 minutes. Avoid during pregnancy.

Dry, sensitive, or mature skin

To a basin of boiling water, add 1 drop each of the essential oils of patchouli, frankincense, and camomile. Cover your head with a towel, close your eyes, and relax into the steam for 5 minutes.

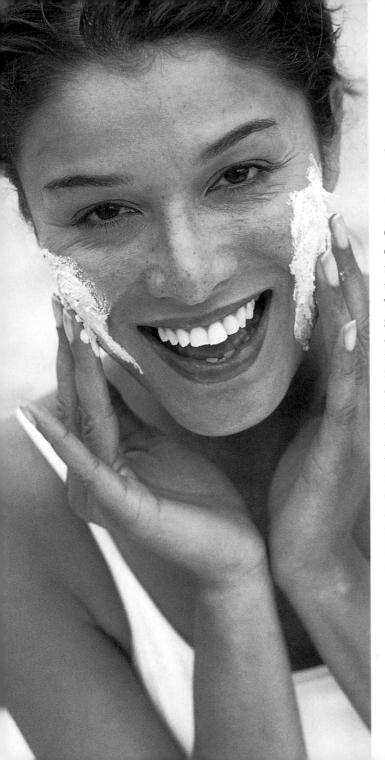

Face masks & packs

Once a week, treat your face to one of these deep-cleansing, skin-smoothening treatments made from pulverized spices, invigorating tropical fruit, and spirit-lifting floral extracts. These Indian facial delights for a silky smooth, glowing complexion and supple skin have been around for thousands of years. As you relax, imagine all impurities dissolving and being flushed away by the pure, clean water that completes these treatments. The turmeric mask is recommended for darker-toned skins, as it imparts a wonderful glow, and is also reputed to slow down the growth of facial hair. Indian women swear by the softening powers of gram flour (milled from the highly nutritious chickpea). Use a gram flour mask regularly over a period of three months for visible improvements. Applied before facial steaming (*see page 25*), a honey mask will allow the hot steam to penetrate skin more effectively.

Turmeric treasure

- 1 tbsp ground turmeric
- 1 tbsp milk
- your dosha-specific cleansing powder

Mix the ground turmeric with enough milk to make a paste. Apply a thin layer over your face. Relax for 10 minutes. Wash off with the cleansing powder for your dosha type (see page 24). Don't use more than once a week unless specified.

Refreshing sandalwood

- 2 tbsp gram flour
- 1 tbsp live natural yogurt
- 6 drops essential oil sandalwood

Mix the flour with enough yogurt to make a paste, then add the oil. Massage over your face, avoiding eyes and mouth. Relax for 10 minutes. Splash off with water.

Gram flour mask

- 2 tbsp gram flour
- a pinch ground turmeric
- 1 tub live natural yogurt
- 2-3 drops lemon or lime juice (oily skin)
- 2-3 drops sweet almond oil (dry skin)

Mix the gram flour, turmeric, and natural yogurt into a paste. Add in either the lemon or lime juice, or sweet almond oil. Smooth over face and neck. Relax for 20 minutes. Splash off with warm water. Repeat 2-3 times a week.

Moisturizing honey mask

- 2 tbsp unpasteurized honey
- 2 tsp freshly squeezed lemon or lime juice

Mix the honey and juice. Pat the mixture on your face and neck using upward, circular movements. Relax for 15 minutes. Rinse off with warm water.

Fruit masks & peels

The natural enzymes in tropical fruits like papaya and pineapple work as gentle exfoliants to remove dead skin cells and revitalize the complexion. Pineapple and papaya are also a rich source of protective antioxidants. Watermelon is a traditional Ayurvedic food used to counteract the pitta heat of high summer; as it refreshes the skin, it clears up blemishes.

Indonesian banana mask

- 2 ripe bananas
- 1 tbsp unpasteurized honey

Blend the bananas and honey into a paste. Pat onto your face and neck. Leave on for 15 minutes. Rinse off with cool water. Repeat every 2-3 days.

Anti-aging avocado mask

- 1 ripe avocado
- 1 tbsp unpasteurized honey
- 2 evening primrose oil capsules
- 1 tbsp rosewater

Mash up the avocado and mix in the honey. Blend in the oil from the capsules. Pat onto your face and neck. Leave on for 20 minutes. Rinse off with cool water or wipe with a cotton ball soaked in rosewater. Use once a week.

Pineapple peel

- ½ peeled and cored pineapple
- 1 tbsp finely ground oatmeal
- 1 cup cool camomile tea

Blend the pineapple in a food processor and combine with the oatmeal. Moisten with enough of the tea to form a paste. Apply to your face and neck, avoiding the eye area. Leave on for 10 minutes. Rinse with cool water.

Clarifying mask

- 1 tbsp yellow mustard seeds
- a handful fresh or dried rose petals

Grind the seeds in a coffee grinder with the petals. Moisten with water to form a thin paste. Apply to your face and neck. Leave on for 20 minutes. Rinse off with cool water. Don't use more often than once a month.

Balinese watermelon mask

- 1 large slice watermelon
- 1 tbsp finely ground oatmeal
- 1 tbsp tamarind water

Blend the flesh of the watermelon in a food processor. Strain the seeds through a sieve. Mix in the oatmeal with the puréed flesh to make a sticky paste. Moisten with a little tamarind water. Pat on your face and neck. Leave on for 15 minutes. Rinse off with hot, then cool water.

Papaya peel

- 1 ripe papaya

Scoop out the papaya flesh and use for another recipe or eat. Cut the skin into two large pieces. Gently massage each one over your face and neck for up to 2 minutes. Avoid the eye area. Rinse off with cool water.

At the Four Seasons Resort on the island of Kuda Huraa in the Maldives, all-natural restorative face masks nourish skin after the cleansing effects of Ayurvedic powders.

Toning waters

After cleansing, apply a refreshing facial toner to close up pores. Cucumber is perhaps nature's finest facial astringent—its pH of 5.48 echoes the skin's own 5.5—and it is valued throughout the tropics to cool sun-parched skin and tighten up pores, especially during the hot summer months. Eau de cologne was the first spice water to become a staple product of European body and beauty care, hailed after its 1709 invention in Köln, Germany, as an invigorating "miracle water." Keep toners in an atomizer in the fridge for a mist of instant freshness.

Lemon grass toner (for oily skin)

- 1 stalk fresh lemon grass
- 1 ginseng tea bag

Chop up the lemon grass. Place in a pan and pour in 2 cups of water. Add the tea bag and bring to the boil. Simmer for 10 minutes. Allow to cool. Strain before using. Refrigerate and use within 3 days.

Rice-water softener

In Indonesia, women regard rice water (the water used to rinse rice before cooking) as a vitamin-rich skin softener. Wash some rice in a bowl and pour off the top layer of water. Gently rinse your face with this cloudy sediment.

Citrus glow

- juice from ½ orange, lemon, or lime
- 1 tbsp rosewater

Dip your fingertips in freshly squeezed orange, lemon, or lime juice. Pat over your cheeks, forehead, chin, and neck. Splash off after 2-3 minutes with water or use a cotton ball soaked in rosewater.

Cucumber cooler

- ½ cucumber
- 1 tbsp fresh coconut water

Juice the whole cucumber. Push the pulp through a fine-mesh sieve to remove any seeds. Blend in a little of the coconut water. Pat on your face. Splash off with water after 2-3 minutes.

Eau de cologne

- 10 tbsp vodka
- 5 drops each essential oils of neroli, bergamot, petitgrain, and geranium
- 3 drops each essential oils of rosemary and orange
- 4 cardamom pods
- 4 cloves
- 2 tbsp spring water

Pour the vodka into a sterilized jar. Drop in the oils and spices. Lid and shake. Leave for 2 days. Add the water. Leave for 1 week. Strain through a coffee filter in a funnel into a sterilized glass bottle. Lid.

Anti-blemish treatments

Refreshing Sandalwood (*see page 27*) is the key Ayurvedic treatment for blemishes, but fenugreek leaves and orange peel offer equally effective alternatives. Blend the sandalwood paste with a little rosewater and, if you have darker skin, add a pinch of ground turmeric. Apply to pimples and blotches overnight. Rinse off with cold water the next morning.

Fenugreek zap

- a handful fenugreek leaves

Grind the leaves using a pestle and mortar. Moisten with enough water to create a paste-like consistency. Apply it to pimples and blackheads. Leave on overnight. Rinse off with warm water the next morning.

Citrus yogurt blitz

- 1 tsp dried orange peel
- 1 tsp live natural yogurt

Pound the peel into a powder with a pestle and mortar. Mix in enough yogurt to make a paste. Apply to spots and acne scars. Leave on for 15 minutes. Splash off with water.

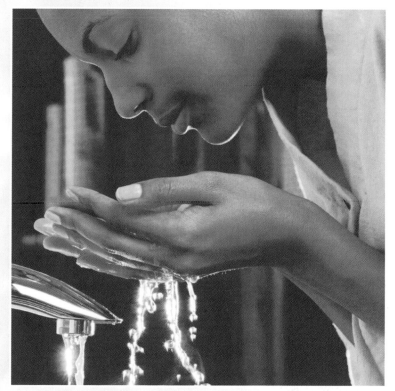

Moisturizing facial oils

Create a moisturizer suited to your dosha type (*see pages 14-15*) and to the fragrances that most appeal to you—your signature facial-oil blend—by mixing up your favorite essential spice and floral oils. Blend the oils in advance and store them in dark-colored, sterilized glass bottles in a cool place for up to three months. Apply the oil to damp skin to help seal in moisture, then just spritz your face during the day with cooling spring water whenever your skin feels parched or in need of rehydration. Make sure that you drink at least eight glasses of spring water—your skin's most natural type of moisturizer—every day.

Vatas

- 1½ tbsp sesame or sweet almond oil
- 10 drops in total essential oils (choose from sandalwood, rose, frankincense, cinnamon, vanilla, or neroli)

Drop the essential oils into the base oil. Shake and apply liberally to damp skin. To rebalance your dosha, rub a little into your third eye area (between your eyebrows).

Pittas

- 1½ tbsp sunflower or sweet almond oil
- 10 drops in total essential oils (choose from ylang ylang, sandalwood, coriander, or rose)

Drop the essential oils into the base oil. Shake and apply to damp skin where required. To rebalance your dosha, rub a little into the center of your chest.

Kaphas

- 1½ tbsp sweet almond oil
- 10 drops in total essential oils (choose from bergamot, cinnamon, frankincense, patchouli)

Drop the essential oils into the base oil. Shake and apply to damp skin sparingly. To rebalance your dosha, rub a little just below your navel.

Super nourishing anti-wrinkle oil

- 1 tbsp sweet almond oil
- 1 tsp sesame oil
- ½ tsp each avocado and wheatgerm oil
- 4 drops essential oil lavender
- 2 drops each essential oils of rose and frankincense
- 1 drop each essential oils of fennel and cypress
- 1 vitamin E capsule

Combine the various oils by shaking them in a dark-colored bottle. Drop in the essential oils. Puncture the vitamin capsule with a pin and squeeze its contents into the bottle. Shake well before using after cleansing last thing at night.

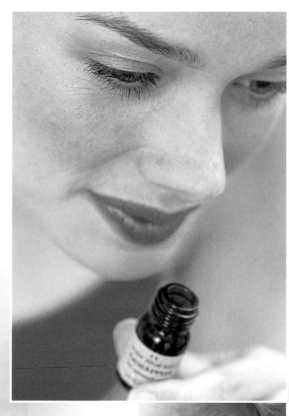

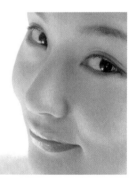

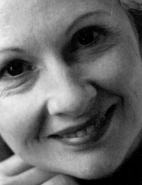

Use the rejuvenescent powers of essential oils to combat aging.

Regenerating facial & footbath

Use this facial as a relaxation ritual to revitalize skin. Set aside one hour once every two weeks. Mix the products in advance and refrigerate. Prepare a pile of clean, warm towels, wash cloths, and cotton balls. Light candles and incense (sandalwood is the best choice). Switch on relaxing music, be it Indians *ragas*, a Balinese gamelan orchestra, or chilled ambient sounds. Ensure the room is warm and that you're wearing something comfortable.

Facial scrub

- 2 tsp ground almonds
- 2 tsp gram flour
- 1 tbsp rosewater

Footbath

- 3 drops each essential oils of lavender and peppermint
- a handful rose petals or dried lavender
- 2 tsp sesame oil

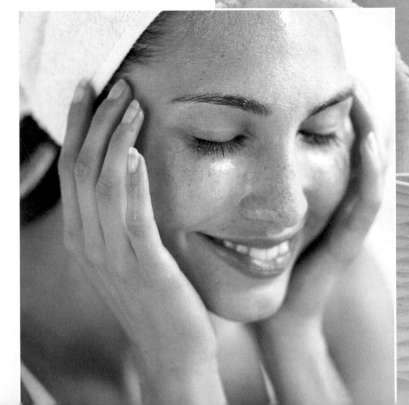

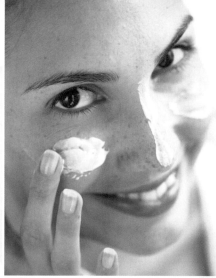

1 Lie on your back, legs relaxed, feet facing outward, arms away from your sides, palms up. Close your eyes. Take deep breaths. Breathe oxygen into areas where there is tension. Exhale aches and pains. Focus on relaxing every part of your body, starting with your toes. Methodically work your way to your scalp, allowing each area to relax in turn. After 10 minutes, open your eyes, wiggle your fingers and toes, roll on one side, and come to sitting position.

2 Remove any make-up and other impurities by following your dosha-specific cleansing routine for face and neck (see page 24). Finish with the Cucumber Cooler or the Lemon Grass Toner (see page 30).

3 Mix the ground almonds, and gram flour with enough rosewater to make a paste. Massage onto your face and neck using circular movements. Do not scrub. Avoid the eye area. Soak a clean wash cloth in hot water to lift away the scrub. Splash off with water. Pat dry. Tone again. Apply the Honey, Banana, or Avocado Masks (see pages 26-29) to your face.

4 To a basin of warm water, add the drops of essential oils and scatter in petals or dried lavender. Soak your feet for 5 minutes. Dry your feet and massage them with warm sesame oil (first stand the bottle in a bowl of hot water).

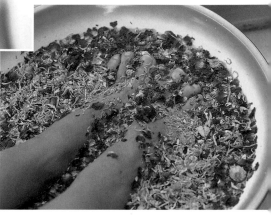

5 Remove the face mask with a warm, wet wash cloth. Pat dry. Tone again. Nourish and rehydrate your skin by boosting the flow of energy to face, neck, and scalp with invigorating natural face-lift massage strokes (see pages 36-37) using the signature moisturizing oil recommended for your dosha type (see page 32).

Inner & outer rejuvenation

Simply relaxing your face with soothing massage strokes can be enough to take off the years and restore inner peace. Start relaxing by stepping back from the world in times of stress to recall a feeling of wellbeing and serenity. Practicing for as little as five minutes a day can make you look radiant and visibly younger. When you're feeling particularly stressed, lie or sit down, close your eyes, and transport yourself back to a time when you felt at one with the world—perhaps lazing on a warm beach, taking a mountain hike, or lying with a baby blissfully asleep on your chest. An inability to de-stress can often cause headaches. Below are treatments to help alleviate such physical signs of stress as well as rejuvenating body, mind, and spirit.

Soothing headache remedy

- 1 tsp turmeric powder
- 1 tsp sweet almond oil

Blend the powder with enough oil to make a smooth paste. Lie back and close your eyes. Massage into your temples and the third-eye area (between your eyebrows). These are powerful *marma* points (energy junctions along the body). Relax for 5 minutes, breathing slowly. Imagine the pain dissolving and being wiped away as you remove any yellow staining afterward with a little almond oil on a cotton ball.

Ayurvedic face-lift

This facial self-massage helps to clear energy blockages and allows the free flow of *prana* (life energy) by activating vital energizing *marma* pressure points on the face, neck, and scalp. This not only gives you clear, glowing skin, but is thought to help develop spiritual awareness. Start by dipping your fingertips in a tiny amount of your dosha-specific facial oil (*see page 32*).

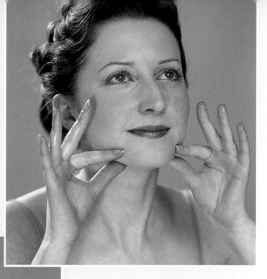

4 Press the area between your forehead and eyebrows with your right thumb. Pinch your eyebrows with your thumbs and index fingers, drawing them outward. Press again at your temples with your index fingers. Repeat 3 times.

1 Start by making upward strokes with your fingers up the front of your neck toward your chin. Start on either side of your trachea, moving your hands around your neck to finish behind your ears.

5 Place your fingertips in the center of your forehead and draw them out to your hairline, pressing at your temples. Repeat 3 times.

2 With thumbs and index fingers touching, place them in the center of your chin, index fingers on top, thumbs underneath. Sweep up and around your jawline. When your fingers reach your ears, briefly press just below your lobes. Repeat 3 times.

6 Rest the fleshy part of your palms over your eye sockets for 30 seconds, without pressing on your eyeballs. Relax and look into complete darkness. Release.

3 Place your ring fingers on both cheekbones where they meet your nose. Draw them out along your cheekbones. Press in at your temples. Repeat 3 times.

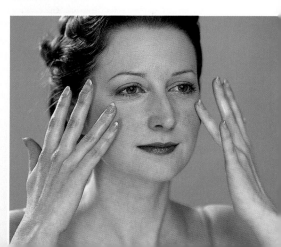

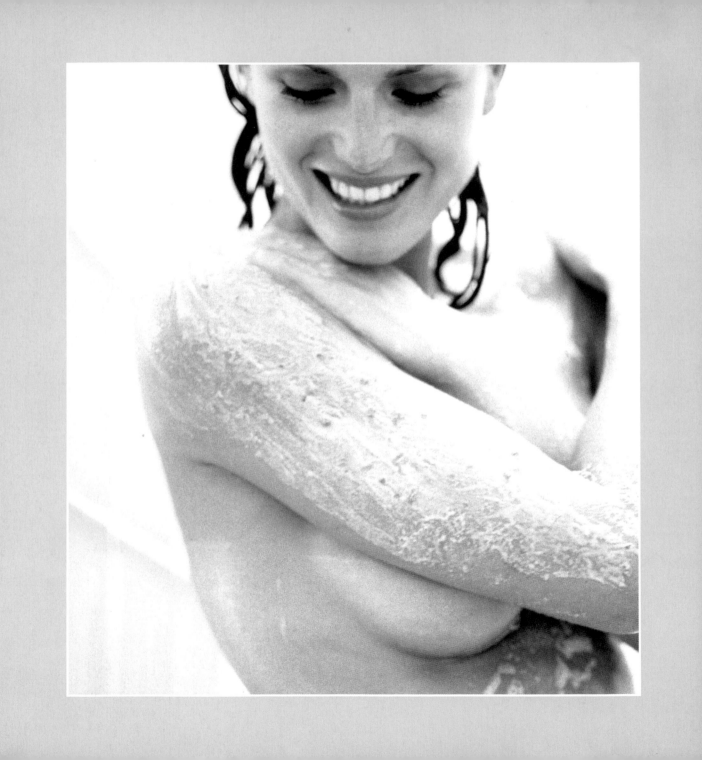

pampering body treats

In the tropical spas of Bali and Thailand, the islands of the Indian Ocean and the Caribbean, lengthy cleansing rituals of two hours or more prepare the body to absorb nourishing moisturizers with exfoliating spice scrubs, body polishes, and deep-cleansing masks that draw out toxins. Any residual tension is smoothed away with massage treatments followed by a smothering of body milks and unguents to condition and contour the body. Some spice rubs take culinary inspiration as their starting point such as the almond *masala* nutrient-rich body scrub created by the Island Spa in the Maldives. Based on the Indian culinary must-have spice powder—*garam masala*—its almond, nutmeg, black pepper, cardamom, and clove leaf ingredients have a warming and balancing effect on the body.

Black pepper & basil exfoliating treatment

This sensuous recipe was created by Luisa Anderson, manager of the lavish Island Spa at the Four Seasons Resort on Kuda Huraa island in the Maldives. Surrounded by sun, sand, and sea, guest spa pavilions have cutaway floorboards so you can gaze down into the limpid depths of the ocean as you receive the treatment. The exfoliation starts with a herb-infused bath, the scented hot water easing away muscular aches and mental fatigue. The body buff is uplifting, warming, cleansing, and imparts physical benefits as well as mental vigor. Prepare the recipe beforehand and finish off the treatment with a soothing shower, especially refreshing after a long journey or a hard day at work.

Caution: Do not perform whole body exfoliation treatments during pregnancy.

Ingredients

- 2 tbsp fine sea salt
- 1½ tsp finely cracked black pepper
- 2 tbsp cold-pressed olive oil or grapeseed oil
- 7 drops essential oil basil
- 4 drops essential oil black pepper
- freshly squeezed juice ½ lemon
- non-perfumed shower gel (optional)
- a handful basil leaves

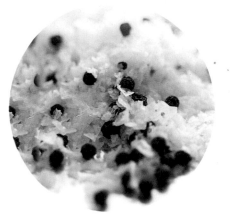

The black pepper in the scrub warms tired muscles by bringing a fresh supply of blood to every body part. The benefits include relaxation, motivation, clear thinking, and physical endurance.

1 Mix the salt and pepper. Add the olive oil, essential oils, and lemon juice. Use more oil or a little shower gel for extra lubrication. Set aside.

2 While you run the bath, infuse the basil in boiling water for 10 minutes. Before stepping in, strain the infusion and stir it into the water. Relax for 20 minutes.

3 Once out of the bath, massage handfuls of the spice scrub over your moistened skin, starting with the soles of your feet and working your way up your legs with large, circular strokes in the direction of your heart.

4 Brush your torso, arms, and neck, concentrating on your buttocks, thighs, and upper arms—those parts of the body that really benefit from invigorating circulation boosts. After 15 minutes, rub off the mix with a warm wet wash cloth.

5 First take a warm, then a cool shower to rinse away the remaining salt and pepper granules and refresh heated skin. After patting your skin dry, apply a hydrating body milk, preferably one containing lemon and basil.

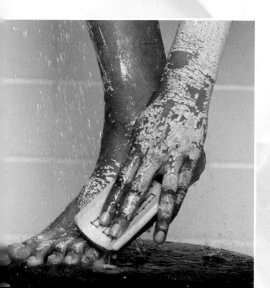

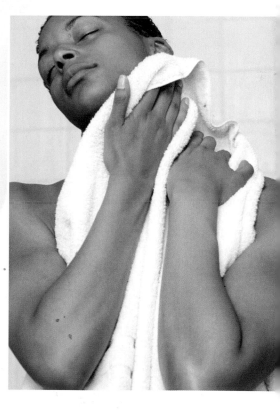

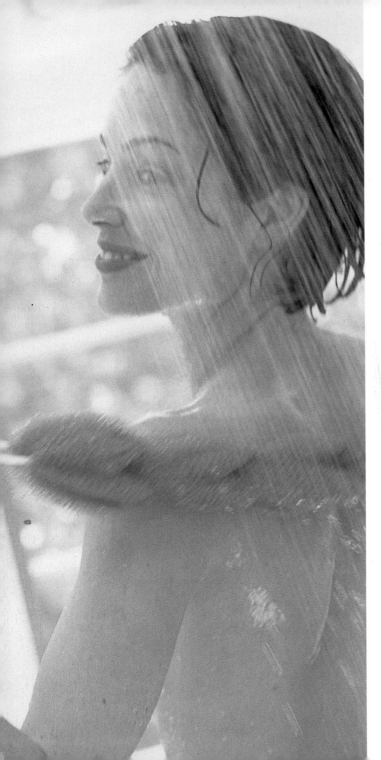

Body mask & scrub

At the Chiva-Som Health Resort in Thailand, the body is exfoliated using papaya, pineapple, and aloe vera. You are then enveloped in banana leaves to keep you warm as your scalp is massaged first with a restorative essential oil, then a mineral-rich hair mud. A rebalancing aromatherapy massage follows.

The Honey and Sesame Scrub recipe is inspired by the Oriental Body Glow treatment on offer at the Oriental Spa in Bangkok, Thailand. This polish leaves skin feeling soft, smooth, hydrated, glowing, and tingling. When the lavender, mint, and sesame are combined with the honey and massaged into damp skin, they remove dead cells and boost circulation to help you feel clean and full of vitality. This is a fantastic emollient pre-massage preparation for all skin types.

Before you start the mask treatment, make sure you have already blended the mask and have a large, clean plastic sheet (available from do-it-yourself stores) and plenty of warm towels at the ready. For the scrub treatment, you will need a loofah or a body brush.

Caution: Do not perform whole body exfoliation treatments during pregnancy.

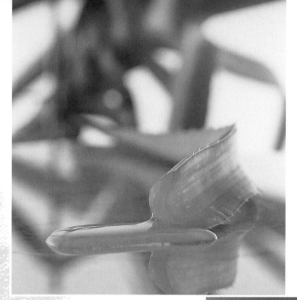

Healing aloe vera gel is derived from the pulpy tissue lining the inner portion of the leaves.

Tropical aloe vera fruit mask

- 1 large, peeled, ripe papaya
- 1 peeled and cored pineapple
- 1 aloe vera leaf
- 1 tube aloe vera gel

Blend the fruit in a food processor. Slice the leaf down the middle, squeeze out its juice, and stir into the fruit paste. Mix in enough gel to make a moist consistency. Set aside. Run a warm bath. Blend 10 drops of your favorite essential oil in 1½ tbsp of base oil and swish a little into the bath before stepping in or use essential oils suited to your dosha (see page 56). Relax for 20 minutes. Pat yourself dry. Apply the mask over your body. Wrap yourself in the plastic sheet, then the towels. Relax for 20 minutes. Take a warm shower without using soap. Apply moisturizer (see pages 60-63) or follow with an aromatherapy massage (see pages 56-57).

Honey & sesame scrub

- 2 tbsp black sesame seeds
- 4 tbsp unpasteurized honey
- a pinch each dried mint and lavender
- 3 drops essential oil lemon grass

Blend all the ingredients into a paste and rub into your body starting with the soles of your feet. Massage your way toward the neck with firm and brisk strokes. Brush the skin with a damp loofah to stimulate circulation and invigorate the skin. After 30 minutes, take a warm shower without using soap to rinse off any excess polish .

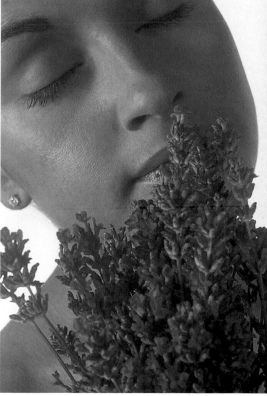

Balinese boreh

Traditionally applied in Balinese villages after a long, back-breaking day to prevent, as well as ease, aches, pains, chills, and fever, this deep-heat treatment is especially restorative for aching feet. Its constituent ginger is strongly antiseptic and restores the flow of chi energy around the body. The intense heat of this treatment is not for the faint-hearted. As well as being part of most Balinese spa menus, it is available at the Shambala Spa within the Parrot Cay Luxury Resort in the Turks and Caicos islands of the Caribbean.

Caution: Do not perform whole body exfoliation treatments during pregnancy.

Ingredients

- 1 tbsp ground sandalwood
- 4 tsp whole ground cloves
- 2 tsp finely grated fresh ginger root
- 1 ground cinnamon stick
- 2 tsp ground coriander seeds
- 1 tsp ground turmeric
- 2 tsp grated nutmeg
- 4 tsp rice powder (baby rice)
- 3-4 tbsp sweet almond oil
- 4-5 roughly grated carrots

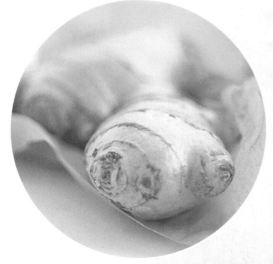

Ginger regenerates skin by stimulating tissue production and detoxifying it from within.

1 Mix the spices with the rice powder. Moisten with enough oil to make a paste. Massage this all over your body up to your neck, paying particular attention to your feet, legs, and any areas with muscular aches.

2 Leave on the rub for 10 minutes for an intense, deep-heat treatment. Give yourself a foot massage while you wait.

3 Massage off the rub with a warm, wet wash cloth. Rub handfuls of grated carrot on your skin to cool and moisturize it. Wipe away before stepping into the bath.

4 Take a Balinese Floral Bath (*see pages 66-67*) before smothering your body in moisturizing body oils and lotions (*see pages 60-63*).

Javanese lulur

Lulur, a body-bath beauty ritual from the royal palaces of central Java, which in the local language means "coating the skin," is the ultimate in pampering, using sweet and spicy powders to polish and soften the body. In use since the 17th century, it was traditionally performed daily for 40 days prior to the nuptial celebration, but today's brides tend to limit its use to the week before their weddings. It is a popular treatment on offer at spas all over Indonesia and Thailand and as far afield as Parrot Cay in the Caribbean. The combination of spices and hand-ground rice make an excellent and aromatic exfoliating body scrub. Apply to skin, especially on flaky areas such as elbows, ankles, and knees.

Caution: Do not perform whole body exfoliation treatments during pregnancy.

Ingredients

- 1 tbsp ground turmeric
- 2 tsp ground sandalwood
- 2 tsp ground ginger
- 2 tbsp rice powder (baby rice)
- 6 drops essential oil jasmine
- 1 tub live natural yogurt
- a handful jasmine, hibiscus, frangipani, lavender, or rose petals

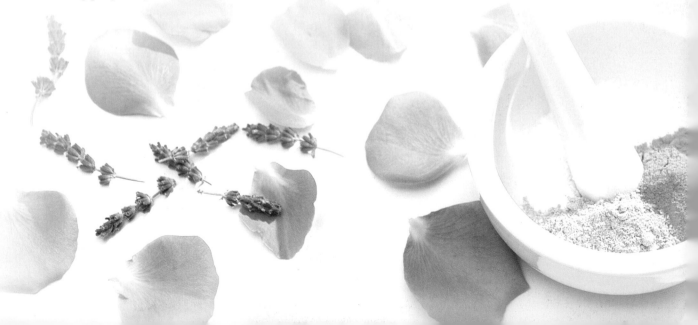

1 Mix the powdered spices and rice together into a paste with a small amount of water until all the ingredients are blended. Stir in the essential oil of jasmine.

2 Apply the paste to your skin. Allow it to dry. Using circular motions to gently exfoliate, rub off the paste before showering. Apply natural yogurt to the skin to cool, moisturize, and soften. Shower off.

3 After showering, treat yourself to a lengthy, luxurious soak in a warm, flower-filled bathtub. Just before immersion, scatter in a handful of petals. Tropical jasmine, hibiscus, and frangipani are traditional choices, but more readily available options include lavender and rose petals, which are equally uplifting. Close your eyes and allow your mind to float away on the floral scent.

Indian ubtan rub

Dating back to Vedic times, this ancient Indian spice formula is arguably the world's earliest cosmetic—promoted to nourish, protect, and beautify skin through the antifungal, antibacterial, and antiperspirant properties of its spices. The rub has been appropriated by Indian brides and grooms, who apply it while reciting holy *mantras* as part of their pre-wedding ceremony. Regardless of your marital status, you, too, will come to value this spice-laden treat for its ability to revitalize, refine, and sweeten skin. Use once a week and, during the treatment, burn light sandalwood incense to heighten the sense of auspiciousness.

Caution: Do not perform whole body exfoliation treatments during pregnancy.

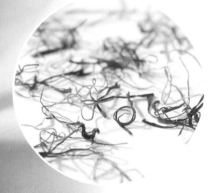

Saffron has a reputation for soothing and softening problematic skin.

Body paste

- 2 tsp ground sandalwood
- 1 tsp grated nutmeg
- 1 tsp ground cumin seeds
- 1 tsp ground yellow mustard seeds
- 2 tsp ground turmeric
- 2-3 crushed saffron strands
- 3 tbsp gram flour
- juice 1 lemon (oily skin)
- 1 tub live natural yogurt (oily skin)
- 1 tbsp milk (dry skin)

Bath soak

- 5-6 tbsp powdered milk
- 1 muslin square or cheesecloth
- 5 drops essential oil sandalwood
- 5 drops essential oil jasmine

1 Mix the ground spices with the gram flour. For oily skin, moisten them into a smooth paste with the lemon juice or yogurt. For drier skin, combine them with a little milk.

2 Rub the paste over your body. Start with your feet, working your way up your legs, hips, and arms in large, circular movements moving toward your heart and circling your joints. Pay attention to areas of rough or uneven skin such as your thighs, buttocks, upper arms, and abdomen.

3 Relax for 5 minutes, protecting surfaces with plastic as the paste can stain. Shower off the paste.

4 Float a muslin bag containing powdered milk scented with sandalwood and jasmine essential oils beneath the faucets as you fill up the bath. Step into this traditional pre-wedding milk bath. Relax for 20 minutes.

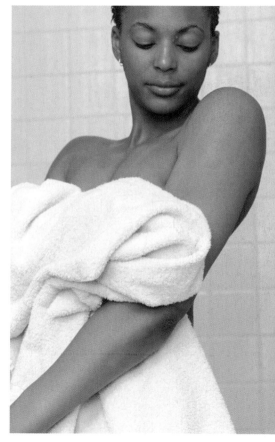

5 Pat skin dry and, while it is still damp, apply an Oriental-scented body lotion. Look for one with ylang ylang, patchouli, or jasmine.

Purifying wrap

Linen sheets soaked in herbs and spices are used to cocoon the body in spas the world over to stimulate the circulatory and lymphatic systems and eliminate toxins. They also soothe overworked muscles, revitalize skin, and enhance the immune system. This treatment is on offer at the Chiva-Som Health Resort in Thailand. As you sip herbal tea (a blend of fresh ginger, camomile, and mint), your body is brushed to encourage the flow of lymph—one of the body's waste-disposal systems—and begin a process of detoxification. You are then wrapped in steaming linen infused with the same mix of spices and herbs. Replicate this at home by using the heat from a steaming bath. Repeat this treatment twice a week to stimulate and detoxify. You will need a a loofah or body brush.

Caution: Avoid this treatment if you are pregnant, suffer from high or low blood pressure, varicose veins or thrombosis, are sensitive to heat, or have a cold or flu.

Ingredients

- ½ sliced cucumber
- 4 tsp grated ginger root
- 3 tsp dried camomile flowers
- 1½ tsp washed mint leaves
- 1 large muslin square or cheesecloth
- 1 tsp unpasteurized honey

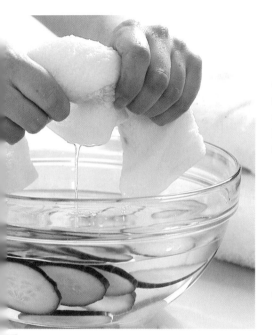

1 Take a few slices of cucumber and place them in a bowl of freshly boiled water. Steep a wash cloth in it for 30 minutes. Remove it and wring out any extra water. Roll it up. Refrigerate for 1 hour before starting the treatment.

2 Pound the ginger into small pieces with a knife handle or a rolling pin.

3 Place a little ginger, camomile, and mint in a teapot. Pour in boiling water. Steep for 5 minutes.

4 Place the remaining ginger, camomile, and mint on the muslin cloth. Tie the top to secure. Run a hot bath, leaving the herbs to steep and the water to cool for 15 minutes. Keep the door closed to ensure that the heat remains trapped in the bathroom.

5 Start to brush the soles of your feet with a loofah or body brush. Work your way up to your neck in circular strokes toward your heart.

6 Strain and sip the tea (sweetened with honey if desired) before soaking in the bath for 20 minutes. Place the wash cloth over your eyes.

7 After the bath, wrap yourself in a warm robe, drink plenty of water, and relax. Rinse and dry the cloth bag to re-use in another bath.

Total detoxification

Like Traditional Chinese Medicine (TCM), Ayurveda places great emphasis on detoxifying regimes to purify the system from within. While the Indian Ayurvedic tradition mainly recommends body oiling and steaming, special diets and herbs are also prescribed, as in TCM. Turmeric and ginger are supportive of the liver, which cleanses the blood by filtering out waste products. Licorice boosts the kidneys, considered in TCM to be the "root of life," the site of chi energy. Detox in the spring to rid your body of winter toxins, and in the fall to strengthen the system.

Caution: Do not detox if you are pregnant or breastfeeding, if you feel ill, are recovering from illness, or have a medical condition. If you have any concerns, consult your doctor.

Body scrub & bath bag

- a handful sea salt
- 1 muslin square or cheesecloth

Vatas: 1 tsp each freshly grated ginger root, cardamom pods, fennel seeds, and 1 cinnamon stick
Pittas: 1 tsp each coriander, cumin, and fennel seeds
Kaphas: 1 tsp each freshly grated ginger root, cloves, and mustard seeds

Detox bath

- 10 drops in total essential oils (choose from frankincense, eucalyptus, vetiver, or juniper)
- 1½ tbsp carrier oil (choose from sweet almond or sesame)
- 1 Chinese licorice or fennel tea bag

Guidelines

- Eat lightly. Choose steamed seasonal vegetables or freshly juiced fruit and vegetables (apple, pomegranate, beetroot, and carrot). Add seeds and grains to meals (millet, barley, and quinoa are cleansing and supportive; sesame and sunflower seeds offer an instant energy push). Spice up your food with turmeric, cumin, cinnamon, saffron, and coriander, as in *kitchari*, the Ayurvedic detox recipe.
- Avoid processed foods, animal products, and dairy except for live natural yogurt. Avoid eating later than 7 p.m.
- Cut out tea, coffee, sugar, and alcohol. Replace them with herbal teas and infusions (Chinese licorice root, peppermint, or fennel).
- Drink at least eight glasses of water a day.
- Take plenty of exercise.

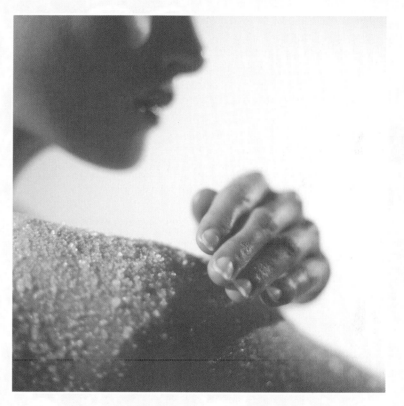

1 In the morning, treat your body to a warm oil massage suited to your dosha (*see pages 14-15*) and dislodge toxins toward their removal sites (for oils and stroke types, *see pages 54-55*). Imagine your stresses melting into the oil along with your body's waste products. After 15 minutes, take a hot shower without scrubbing off all the oil.

2 Massage the sea salt into your skin using large, sweeping, circular strokes toward your heart. Work your way up your legs, arms, and torso to reach your neck.

 Fill up the tub for your spice-infused hot bath. Spoon your dosha-specific spices into the muslin square and tie to leave. Place under the running hot water faucet. Relax in the bath for at least 10 minutes, focusing on your breathing. Drain the water from your bathtub.

4 In the evening, run another hot bath. Add the essential oils to the carrier oil. Shake. Pour into the bathwater. Step in. Sip the tea. Relax briefly (vatas), follow with a cool shower (pittas), or soak at length (kaphas).

5 Before going to bed, treat your scalp, the soles of your feet, and any areas of tension to a warm, sesame oil massage.

Ayurvedic self-massage

Ayurvedic massage practice works to free up the key energy centers of the body; the practice of *abhyanga* (applying oil to the skin) also enhances lymph activity and blood circulation, enabling toxins to pass through the skin's surface. It noticeably improves your mental and physical wellbeing as well as giving you great skin! Work this 20-minute, self-massage into part of your morning routine three days a week if you are a vata. Pittas and kaphas benefit from making it a weekly treat (to assess your dosha type, *see pages 14-15*).

Caution: Avoid if you have a fever, high blood pressure, or skin problems.

Burning oils

Vatas: 3-4 drops in total essential oils (choose from ylang ylang and patchouli)
Pittas: 3-4 drops in total essential oils (choose from saffron, jasmine, rose, and sandalwood)
Kaphas: 3-4 drops in total essential oils (choose from frankincense and cedar)

Massage oils

Vatas: 1½ tbsp sesame oil
Pittas: 1½ tbsp sunflower or coconut oil
Kaphas: 1½ tbsp mustard oil

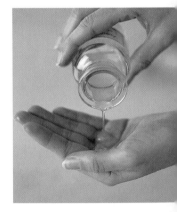

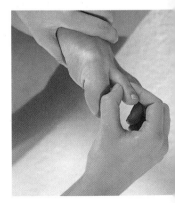

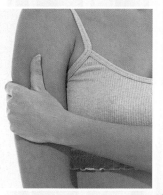

4 Massage both buttocks. Rest both hands on your pelvis. Make small, circular, clockwise movements just below your navel, at your solar plexus, and around your abdomen. Massage your chest and shoulders using large, rhythmic strokes. Rest your hands over the center of your chest. Reaching behind, rub your back with the oil. Squeeze any knotted muscles.

5 Rub up and down the sides of your neck. Lightly rest your palms over the center of your throat. Massage it and your face using delicate upward and outward movements over the jawline, cheeks, and forehead. Rest your thumbs in prayer position over your third-eye area for a few breaths.

6 Oil your scalp, making small circles with the tips of your fingers from your hairline down the back of your neck. Rest your palms on the crown of your head. Relax for 5 minutes. Shower or bathe, without washing off all the oil.

1 Start to burn the essential oils suited to your dosha type in an oil burner. Select the appropriate massage oil and strokes: gentle (vatas), moderate (pittas), and deeply vigorous (kaphas). Pour some massage oil on your hands. Rub it between both palms to warm it. Work over your left foot in flowing, circular strokes, tapping the sole. Devote time to each toe, pulling away at each tip. Repeat on your right foot.

2 Work up from your ankle to your knee on each leg. Massage both thighs. Use kneading movements over fleshy areas and rounded circles around ankle and knee joints.

3 Massage your left hand, pulling off at the fingertips. Work your left arm and circle your elbow, wrist, and shoulder joints. Repeat on your right hand and arm.

Aromatherapy self-massage

Scented massage lotions concocted from essential oils add an element of luxury to any massage as the oils travel to the limbic (emotional) part of the brain within seconds. The essential oils extracted from spices are traditionally regarded as warming and invigorating, while those obtained from tropical flowers tend to be soothingly uplifting. Choose those scents that most appeal to you, those that have the desired effect on body and mind, or those that bring your dosha into balance. Combine the essential oils with a base (or carrier) oil—try sweet almond or sunflower—before starting this calming sequence.

Caution: Avoid if you have a fever, high blood pressure, or skin problems. If you are pregnant or breastfeeding, consult blending advice first (*see page 61*).

Choosing the right essential oils

Soothing scents: frankincense, lavender, sandalwood.
Healing scents: jasmine, rose.
Aphrodisiac scents: patchouli, jasmine, ylang ylang.
Meditative scents: sandalwood, rose, holy basil (*tulsi*), frankincense.

Dosha-specific scents

Add up to 10 drops in total of these essential oils to 1½ tbsp of your basic massage oil (*see page 54*) according to your dosha type:

Vatas: frankincense, basil, cinnamon, sandalwood, rose, jasmine, vanilla, or patchouli.

Pittas: sandalwood, rose, jasmine, lavender, vanilla, geranium, or lemon grass.
Kaphas: cinnamon, patchouli, cedarwood, frankincense, myrrh, or eucalyptus.

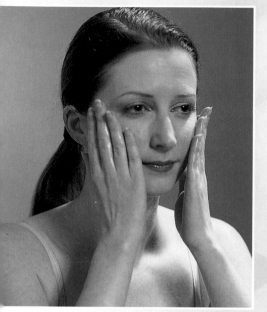

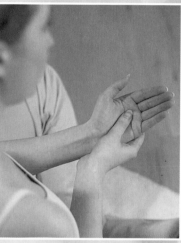

3 Float your right hand down the length of your left arm. When you get to your left hand, cup it in your fingers. Using your right thumb, make short, sliding strokes over your left palm. Repeat on the other arm and hand.

4 Massage your stomach clockwise lifting one hand over the other.

1 Sit cross-legged. Warm the oil between your palms. Circle your cheeks with gentle, warming strokes using your fingers and palms.

2 With your right hand, squeeze and release the muscles down the left side of your neck and across your shoulder blades. Repeat on the other side.

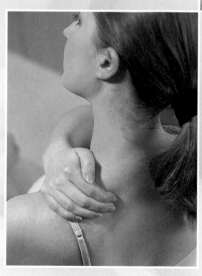

5 Place your hands on your waist at either side of your spine. Move them down your lower back, over your hips, and up and around back to the starting point. Repeat 3 times.

6 Finish by stroking both thumbs up the sole of your left foot and out in a T-shape. Repeat 6 times on both soles. Sandwich each foot in turn between both your hands for 2 minutes.

Reviving self-massage

As you follow this stimulating massage sequence, bring your attention to each part of the body you pass over, breathing vitality into the area and breathing out tension. Before you start the sequence, blend 1½ tablespoons of the base or carrier oil (*see page 56*) with up to 10 drops (in total) of the appropriate essential oils (*see below*) to revive and stimulate body and mind .

Caution: Avoid if you have a fever, high blood pressure, or skin problems. If you are pregnant or breastfeeding, consult blending advice first (*see page 61*).

Choosing uplifting essential oils

Purifying scents: basil, peppermint, eucalyptus.
Fiery scents: cardamom, clove, fennel, ginger.
Stimulating scents: ginger, black pepper, coriander.
Mind-clarifying scents: grapefruit, lemon, juniper.

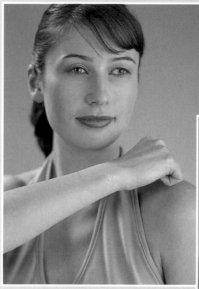

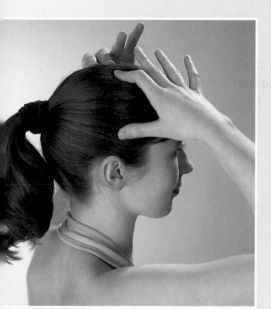

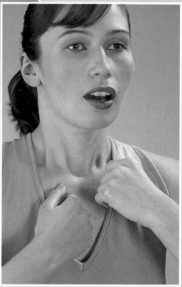

1 Stand up. Tap your fingertips lightly over your scalp from front to back.

2 Making a loose fist with your right hand, pummel over your shoulder on your left side. Repeat with your left fist on your right shoulder.

3 Pour a little oil into your palm and warm it between your hands. Briskly sweep your right hand down your left arm (from your shoulder to your fingertips), pulling off at the tips with an energizing shake of your wrist. Repeat several times. Switch to your left hand on your right arm.

4 Make kneading movements with your right hand down the left side of your neck, across your shoulder and down your upper arm. Repeat on your right side.

5 Pummel your buttocks with soft, loose fists. Using the sides of your hands, bounce them up and down over the fronts and sides of your thighs in a chopping motion.

6 Pummel your chest with soft, loose fists, letting out an "aaahhh" cry.

Body oils & lotions

Replenish skin after an exfoliation or a soothing bath treatment with nutritive body oils and lotions. Choose warming balms enriched with spices, those used during Indonesia's rainy season, during the winter, or at dawn. Cooling lotions come into their own at sunset or during the intense heat of high summer.

Caution: If pregnant and breastfeeding, consult blending advice first (*see opposite*).

Balinese spice oil

- 1½ tbsp coconut oil
- 3 drops each essential oils of fennel, ginger, and vetiver
- 1 drop essential oil of cinnamon or clove (optional)

Balinese santi oil

- 1½ tbsp coconut oil
- 2 drops each essential oils of lemon, petitgrain, nutmeg, vetiver, and patchouli

Refreshing vanilla moisturizer

- 2 tbsp jojoba
- 10 g (⅓ oz) beeswax
- 3 tbsp coconut oil
- 4 tsp rosewater
- 3 drops each essential oils of sandalwood and frankincense
- 2 drops vanilla essence

Melt the jojoba, wax, and coconut oil in a bowl over a pan of boiling water, stirring continuously. Remove the bowl from the heat. Mix in a few drops of rosewater, stirring until it blends as the cream cools. Mix in the essential oils and vanilla essence. Spoon into a sterilized dark glass jar and seal. Refrigerate before using.

Repair balm

After exposing your skin to blistering heat or a day in the sun, drench skin in the refreshing, skin-protecting lotion below. Massage over your body, hands, and face. Relax for 20 minutes while giving yourself a foot or scalp massage. Rub off the excess lotion with a damp wash cloth.

Aloe vera & cucumber lotion

- 1 aloe vera leaf
- 1 cucumber
- 1 tube aloe vera gel
- 2 drops essential oil camomile

Split the aloe vera leaf down the center. Squeeze out its juice with a spoon. Chop up the cucumber (keeping the skin on) and blend in a food processor. Push the pulp through a sieve to remove any large seeds. Stir into the aloe juice. If necessary, add a generous squeeze of gel. Blend in the essential oil well.

Blending essential oils

Essential oils are too concentrated to be applied straight on the skin in their undiluted form. They should be mixed with a carrier or base oil (such as sweet almond, apricot kernel, sunflower, and soya) before use in the following proportions:

Normal dilution

- To 1½ tbsp of base or carrier oil, add 10 drops (in total) of essential oils

Low dilution (for sensitive skin, during pregnancy, and while breastfeeding)

- To 1½ tbsp of base or carrier oil, add 5 drops of essential oils

Use gentle essential oils like rose, sandalwood, frankincense, citrus oils, lavender, camomile, and geranium.

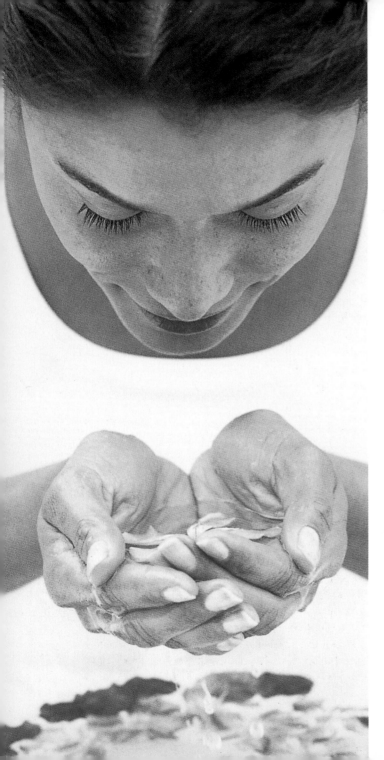

Floral indulgence

The most luxurious way of maximizing the benefits of the floral baths that epitomize the luxury spas of Asia is to subsequently anoint your body with flower-scented milks and oils. Slip into something comfortable, like a rich, subtly scented body cream or oil. All these products nourish, hydrate, and rejuvenate the skin. For best results, apply to warm damp skin after taking a shower or bath. Flower fragrances exercise a uniquely uplifting aromatherapy effect on the mind and the spirit: a secret long-recognized in religious ceremonies, from the jasmine-flower offerings in Buddhist and Hindu temples to floral altarpieces in Christian churches. Surround yourself with these symbols of mystery and romance by using floral unguents on special, pampering days.

Caution: If pregnant or breastfeeding, consult blending advice first (*see page 61*).

Body lotion

- 10 g (⅓ oz) beeswax
- 10 g (⅓ oz) cocoa butter
- 3 tbsp sweet almond oil
- 7 tsp rosewater or orange blossom water
- 2 drops each essential oils of jasmine and rose
- 1 drop vanilla essence

Melt the beeswax, cocoa butter, and oil in a bowl over a pan of boiling water, stirring continuously. Remove from heat. Mix in the flower water a few drops at a time, stirring until the mixture combines together as the cream cools. Mix in the essential oils and vanilla essence. Spoon into a sterilized dark glass jar and seal. Refrigerate.

Body oil

- 1½ tbsp sweet almond oil
- 10 drops in total essential oils (choose from ylang ylang, geranium, lavender, jasmine, rose, or neroli)

Blend the flower essences into the almond oil, varying the proportions of the mix to reflect your mood.

Uplifting visualization

As you smooth a floral oil or lotion over your body, visualize a spiritually elevating color in your mind's eye: orange, for example, counters lethargy or tiredness. Starting to apply the lotion or the oil at your toes, imagine the color seeping up through your limbs to suffuse every part of you. Pause every few strokes and feel your body becoming warmer and tingling. Each time you exhale, imagine that the color is evaporating with your breath and taking with it all your mental fatigue. Once you have covered every part of your body, pause to take in how awake, alert, and refreshed you feel.

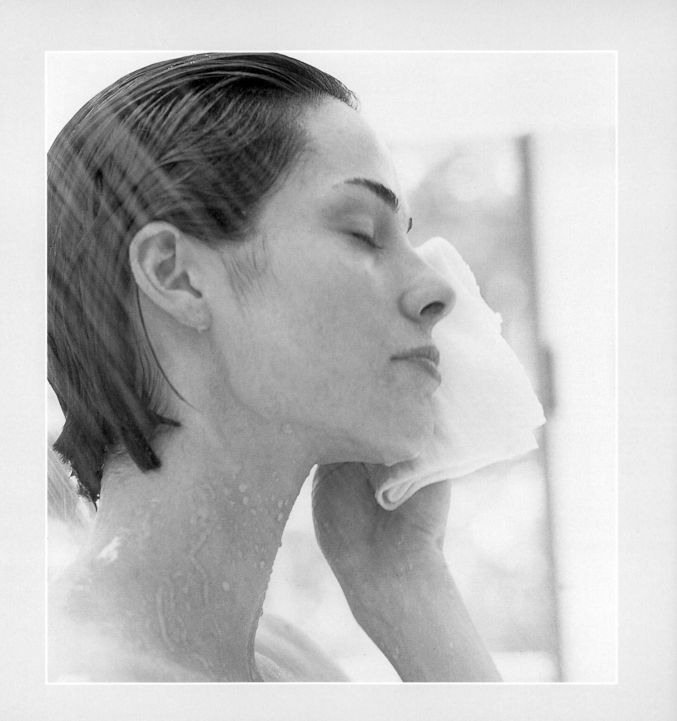

bath & shower delights

Water has been worshipped for its cleansing, healing, and life-giving powers in all its forms since the beginning of time—as ice, mist, steam, snow and, most common of all, as running currents. In the East and West, natural hot springs are pilgrimage sites and wells and springs have been adopted as sources of spiritual wellbeing. Today, spas offer a variety of treatments that involve being sprayed, splashed, rubbed, wrapped, and immersed in water, purifying salts, clays, algae, and other detoxifying substances. The results are amazing—a cleansed, toned body and a clarified mind. Replicate the healing water practices of Java, Japan, Bali, or Morocco by treating yourself to the flower, honey, seaweed, salt, milk, and mud treatments that follow.

Balinese floral bath

Infused with tropical flowers and the essential oils of spices and herbs, a traditional Balinese floral bath is the treatment of choice to end many body-pampering sessions at the world's top spa resorts such as Chiva-Som in Thailand. It is especially welcome after a Balinese massage during which two masseurs work in synchrony, stretching, rolling, and pressing your flesh until it becomes as soft and yielding as butter. Different-hued jasmine petals strewn over water are thought to rebalance the chakra colors they echo. While you relax, sip a herbal tea known as health-giving *Jamu* in Indonesia.

Caution: Use only gentle essential oils (*see page 61*) while pregnant or breastfeeding.

Balinese bath oil

- 1½ tbsp coconut oil
- 7 drops in total essential oils (choose from orange, mandarin, neroli, petitgrain, lemon, and grapefruit)
- 2 drops vanilla essence

Blend the essential oils that most appeal to you into the coconut base oil. Stir in the vanilla essence.

Aphrodisiac bath oil

- 1½ tbsp sweet almond oil
- 10 drops in total essential oils (choose from jasmine, ylang ylang, patchouli, clary sage, and sandalwood)

Drop the essential oils that most appeal to you into the sweet almond base oil.

Sensual dusting powder

- 1 tbsp dried rose petals
- 8 tbsp cornstarch
- 3 drops each essential oils of rose and jasmine

Pound the rose petals into a powder using a pestle and mortar. Place them in a large jar with the cornstarch and lid. Shake to combine. Drop in the essential oils. Shake well to distribute. Store in a cool, dark place.

1 Run a deep, warm bath. Surround the bath with nightlights or scented candles. Turn off other light sources. Scatter in a handful of heady-scented petals such as rose, jasmine, ylang ylang, patchouli, hibiscus, or frangipani.

2 Swish either the Balinese or the Aphrodisiac Bath Oil into the water. Step in.

3 Close your eyes. Relax in the water for 20 minutes or more. To prevent your face from overheating, mist it with an atomizer filled with chilled rosewater or, as an alternative, orange blossom, rose geranium, or lavender water.

4 After the bath, apply a floral Body Lotion or Oil (see page 63) to damp skin. Once dry, shake on the Sensual Dusting Powder. Wrap yourself in a robe, drink a glass of spring water, and lie down to relax for 20 minutes.

Japanese bath

In Japan, the act of bathing is as much a time for peace, solitude, and reflection as it is an opportunity to cleanse the body. It derives from the ritual use of numerous natural hot springs—*onsen*—dotting the Japanese countryside. One first scrubs outside the bath, then steps in to soak in the intensely hot water, feeling aches and pains ease away with the heat. You can recreate the effect of a natural hot spring by adding mineral salts to your bath or, to help ward off winter chills, try a bath bag filled with natural warming spices. After a hot bath, give yourself an acupressure foot massage (*see pages 84-85*). You will need a detachable shower head (or a traditional bamboo cup), a scrub mitt, seaweed soap, and a selection of seasonal flower petals.

Caution: Do not take very hot baths if you are pregnant, suffering from high blood pressure, heart, or vascular problems. Do not use Epsom salts if pregnant. Use only gentle essential oils (*see pages 60-61*) while pregnant or breastfeeding.

Mineral bath salts

- 8 tbsp Epsom salts
- 4 tbsp sea salt
- 3 drops each essential oils of pine and cedarwood

Mix the salts together and spoon into a large jar. Drop the essential oils in and shake well to distribute evenly. Let stand for 1 week in a cool, dark place before use.

Winter bath bag

- ½ freshly sliced lemon
- grated peel (1 mandarin orange)
- 1 tbsp grated ginger root
- 1 muslin square or cheesecloth

Tie up all the ingredients in the square of muslin. Add to the bath before running the water.

Japanese incense

To boost the contemplative mood of the room, light some incense. The five basic ingredients of traditional Japanese incense—aloeswood, clove, sandalwood, turmeric, and borneol —were originally set out in the Buddhist *Sutras*, or holy writings. Japanese incense (*senko*) sticks nowadays also contain spices such as cinnamon bark, myrrh, star anise, licorice root, and ginger, bound together without any artificial ingredients. Japanese incense gives off a light scent that enhances, refreshes, and purifies body and mind, brings alertness and peace to a hectic lifestyle, and provides comfort in solitude.

1   Fill up the bath with very hot water, making it as deep as possible. Add in the Mineral Bath Salts or the Winter Bath Bag. Shut the bathroom door to trap the steam.

2   Step into the shower. Vigorously scrub your body with the mitt and the seaweed soap. Rinse off.

3   Scatter into the bath handfuls of whatever seasonal flowers are available (i.e. traditional cherry blossom in spring or rose petals in summer). Soak in the hot water for 10 minutes.

4   Step out of the bath and wash again with the scrub mitt and seaweed soap. Splash off with cool water.

5   Step into the hot bath once again for a second relaxing 10-minute soak. Feel any residual mental tension melting away into the heat along with any lingering physical aches and pains. Climb out of the bath. Wrap yourself in a robe, lie down, and sip a glass of spring water.

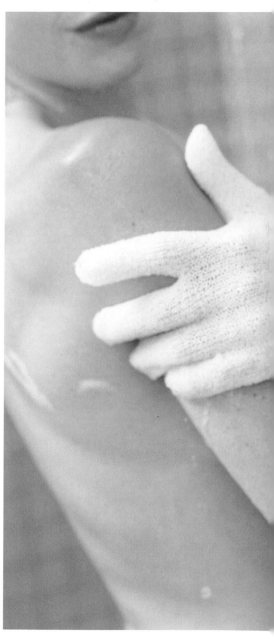

Mandi susu

Hundreds of years ago, in the Indonesian court palaces of Central Java, princesses bathed in spice-infused milk and oils using age-old recipes passed down through the generations. An eternal youth elixir made from milk and honey was also rendered famous by Cleopatra, Queen of Egypt. We offer two bathing rituals here—the first based on the sensational combination of dairy milk and honey, the second on the soothing blend of coconut milk and vanilla. Drench your skin in these sweet-smelling potions and revel in the intoxicating softness.

Caution: Do not take very hot baths if you are pregnant, suffering from high blood pressure, heart, or vascular problems.

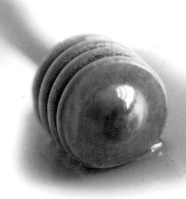

Milk & honey soak

- 5 tbsp powdered milk
- 5 tbsp cornstarch
- 1 tbsp unpasteurized honey
- 10 drops in total essential oils (choose from orange, bergamot, petitgrain, and neroli)

Mix the powdered ingredients with the honey. Moisten with 2 cups of water and stir in the essential oils. Pour into a warm bath. Swish around before stepping in.

Milk & flower bath

- a handful rose petals or jasmine flowers
- body milk of your choice

Apply the Honey and Sesame Scrub (*see page 43*) to dry skin. Shower off after 20 minutes. Avoid using soap. Run a bath. Stir in the Milk and Honey Soak. Throw in a handful of petals or flowers. Relax for 20-30 minutes. Pat yourself dry. Massage the body milk on damp skin.

Vanilla & coconut milk bath

- 1 coconut
- 1 vanilla pod

Après-bain coconut oil

- 1½ tbsp coconut oil
- 5 drops each essential oils of vanilla and lavender

1 Split the coconut in two. Extract and grate the flesh. Cover with warm water. Blend in a food processor and pour into a sieve. With the back of a spoon, press to extract the coconut milk, leaving the grated flesh in the sieve. Set aside.

2 Brush areas of dry skin with the coconut husk to stimulate circulation and exfoliate. Massage the coconut flesh over your body. Leave on for 5 minutes. Wipe away with a warm, wet wash cloth.

3 Fill a bath, placing a vanilla pod in the water as you let the faucets run. Before stepping in, pour in the coconut milk that you extracted earlier. Swish to distribute well. Now blend the essential oils into the coconut base oil. Soak and relax in the bath for 20 minutes. Pat dry. Massage the Aprés-bain Coconut Oil onto damp skin.

Ocean bath

Thalassotherapy treatments ease aches and pains and detoxify the body by boosting circulation and inducing toxin-releasing perspiration. Highly nutritious marine algae condition and rebalance skin through the 103 vitamins, minerals, and organic compounds they contain. As you relax with the body wrap, or soak in the salt bath, play a CD of sea sounds to help your mind gain a sense of widened perspective and infinite horizons. You will need gauze rolls, a large foil sheet (available from camping and outdoor stores), and warm towels for the seaweed wrap. If you feel too lazy to make your own, choose one of the many seaweed gels, muds, masks, and baths available from beauty stores, spas, and drug stores.

Caution: Do not use seaweed if allergic to iodine. Avoid salt scrubs and baths if you are pregnant, suffer from heart disease, or have high blood pressure.

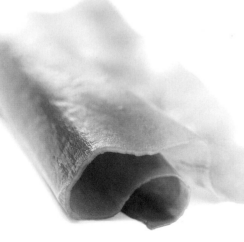

Sea salt scrub

- 10 tbsp sea salt
- 5 drops each essential oils of ginger and mandarin

Dissolve the salt in 10 tablespoons of water. Blend the essential oils. Mix well.

Marine bath

- 10 tbsp sea salt
- 2 freshly sliced limes

Seaweed wrap

- 2 large strips *kombu* or *nori* seaweed
- 6 tbsp dried sage
- 6 tbsp dried mint
- 6 6-in (15-cm) gauze rolls

Heat the strips and herbs in a pan of water. Cover and simmer gently for 20 minutes. Strain. Infuse the gauze rolls in the seaweed liquid until cool.

1 Rub handfuls of the Sea Salt Scrub over your body to exfoliate and stimulate the skin. Starting at the neck, work your way down your torso, arms, and legs using large, circular movements in the direction of your heart. Follow with a cool shower.

2 Wrap the seaweed-soaked gauze around your thighs, buttocks, upper arms, and abdomen. Also cover areas with burst capillaries or visible surface veins.

3 Wrap yourself in the foil sheet, then the warm towels. Lie down and relax for 20 minutes. Remove the strips and discard.

4 Run a warm bath. Add the salt and the limes. Relax for 10 minutes.

5 Take a cool shower and thoroughly rinse off any traces of salt to prevent any skin irritation. Moisturize clean skin with a citrus-scented body oil or lotion.

Moroccan mud bath

This cleansing ritual depends on the purifying properties of steam, mud, peat, and clay to draw out toxins and let skin absorb a complex blend of organic compounds essential for good health. The range of vitamins, minerals, trace elements, amino acids, and enzymes in a particular type of mud varies depending on the region of origin. Austrian Neydharting mud and liquid peat extract are greatly valued in European spas; so, too, is bentonite, the fine French green clay. Products from the Dead Sea, *rhassoul* mud from the Atlas mountains of Morocco, and volcanic Thai mud have likewise been treasured in indigenous body and hair treatments for centuries. A traditional Moroccan *rhassoul* treatment involves covering yourself with the appropriate face and body muds, then relaxing in herbal-scented steam, while you perspire, rubbing in the mud so its water-soluble ingredients can penetrate the skin more effectively. For this treatment, you will need a chair with an old sheet or towel over it.

Caution: Do not use if you are pregnant, suffering from heart disease, or have high blood pressure.

Turmeric is a time-tested beauty aid that not only gives natural gloss, royal glow, and luster, but also imparts vigor and youthful vitality to the entire body.

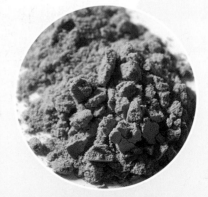

Body clay

- 4 tbsp fuller's earth, kaolin, green clay or, best of all, *rhassoul* mud
- 1 tsp ground turmeric
- 4 tbsp rosewater or orange blossom water
- 6 drops essential oil ylang ylang

Mix the clay and turmeric. Moisten to a paste-like consistency with the flower water. Blend in the essential oil well.

Facial clay

- 2 tbsp kaolin (for normal and oily skin)
- 2 tbsp green clay (for dry and sensitive skin)
- 1 tsp unpasteurized honey
- 1 tsp aloe vera gel
- 1 fennel tea bag

Mix the clay, honey, and aloe vera gel. Moisten to a paste-like consistency with cooled fennel tea.

1 Prepare the Body and Facial Clays, or have a ready-mix selection of store-bought muds suitable for your skin type (available from any health food store).

2 Run a dangerously hot bath (don't worry—you won't be stepping in). Keep the bathroom door closed to trap in steam. Burn 1-2 drops of the essential oils of juniper, cypress, and rosemary in an oil burner or place in a bowl of steaming water.

3 Smear your body with the Body Clay. Apply the Facial Clay, avoiding the eye and mouth area. Relax on the chair. As you perspire, rub the mud over your body to boost circulation. Breathe in the awakening scents of the essential oils.

4 After 15 minutes, take a shower. Gradually reduce the temperature of the water so you finish with a cool blast to close up pores.

5 Pat yourself dry. Give yourself a massage with a body oil or lotion of your choice. Wrap yourself in a robe, lie down, and sip a cooling glass of spring water.

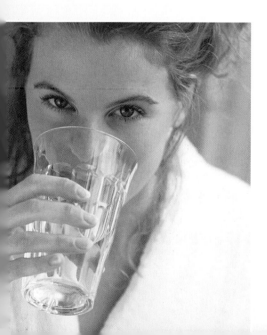

Anti-cellulite hydromassage

Body-contouring hydrotherapy treatments are great for firming up uneven, flabby areas with poor muscle tone. The massage motion of this water-based treatment stimulates circulation and encourages the breakdown of stored toxins as the skin absorbs the beneficial marine and plant extracts in the wraps and the aromatherapy baths. Use this treatment twice weekly for three weeks. You will need a detachable shower head, Sea Salt Scrub (*see page 72*), six 6-in (15-cm) gauze rolls, a large foil sheet (available from camping and outdoors stores), and warm towels.

Caution: Do not use if you are pregnant, suffering from heart disease, or have high blood pressure.

Anti-cellulite massage oil

- 1½ tbsp sesame oil
- 5 drops essential oil rosemary
- 3 drops essential oil lavender
- 2 drops essential oil juniper

Mix the essential oils into the sesame oil.

Skin-reviving bath oil

- 1½ tbsp sesame oil
- 5 drops essential oil lemon grass
- 4 drops essential oil coriander
- 1 drop essential oil clove (optional)

Mix the essential oils into the sesame oil.

Spice-scented towels

- 2 tbsp dried rose petals
- 1 tbsp dried lavender
- 2 crushed cinnamon sticks
- 1 tbsp crushed cloves
- 1 tsp crushed coriander seeds
- 1 tsp crushed cumin seeds
- 1 tsp ground orris root
- 1 tsp salt

Combine all the ingredients in a large bowl, stirring well. Cut a large square of muslin or cheesecloth into several CD-sized squares. Spoon some of the mixture into each square. Secure either with ribbon or raffia. Place the sweetly scented linen bags between your towels to give them a wonderful fragrance.

1 Blend 4 tablespoons of the Sea Salt Scrub into a paste with a little water. Starting with the soles of your feet, massage it all the way up to your neck using firm, circular, and upward movements. Shower off.

2 Rub the Anti-cellulite Massage Oil over your hips, abdomen, and thighs using firm, kneading movements to lift and squeeze your skin. Rotate your knuckles over the same areas and finish with flowing, upward strokes.

3 Wrap these areas with gauze strips. Cover yourself with the foil sheet and warm towels. Relax for 20 minutes. Remove and discard the strips.

4 Run a bath. Swish in the Skin-reviving Bath Oil before stepping in. Relax for 20 minutes as you sip iced lemon grass tea.

5 Before you step out of the bath, direct jets of warm, then cold water at your target areas—thighs, buttocks, and abdomen—using the shower head, making large, then small circles with the spray.

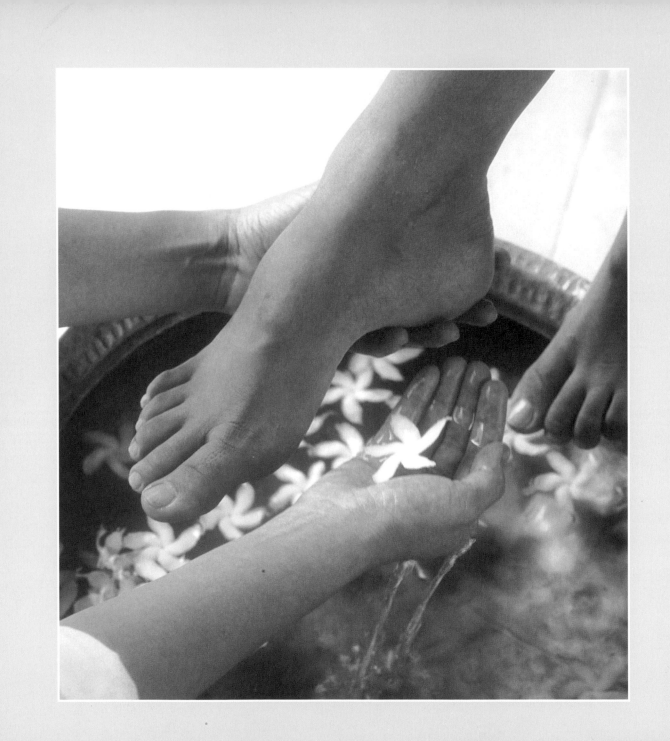

spicy thrills for hands & feet

Beauty treatments for the feet ground the body in similar ways to the practices of yoga and t'ai chi, while manicures and hand massages release overall tension, allowing you to stand tall. Aligning yourself in this way improves posture and restores the free flow of energy through your entire system. The hands and feet are sites of powerful pressure points connecting every part of your body via meridians, or energy channels, so stimulating these vital points with a weekly manicure or pedicure gives you a total workout. Regularly massage your hands and feet after giving yourself a manicure or pedicure. Add spices to these treatments for their powerfully antiseptic and antifungal properties and to stimulate blood flow to the extremities.

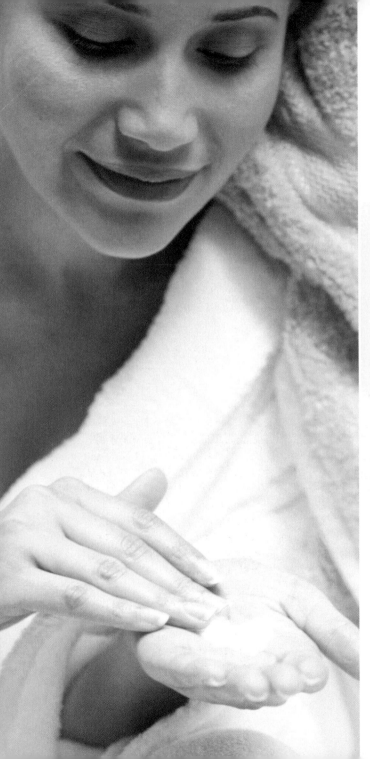

Deep-conditioning hand massage

This massage for the hands using a deeply penetrating, aromatic cream involves working on acupressure points to rebalance energy levels and promote relaxation. Use it every time you give yourself a manicure (*see pages 82-83*) or whenever your hands ache from working at the keyboard or performing other repetitive tasks. Accompany this treatment with reviving and mobilizing hand and wrist exercises (*see page 82*). For ultra supple hands, apply the scented Rich Hand Cream last thing at night before slipping on a pair of cotton gloves. Wear them as you sleep to intensify the penetrating powers of the balm. By morning, your hands will feel luxuriously soft and smooth.

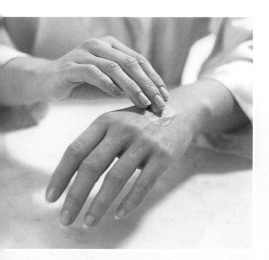

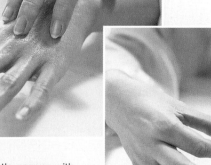

Rich hand cream

- 7 g (¼ oz) beeswax
- 15 g (½ oz) cocoa butter
- 2 tbsp sweet almond oil
- 1 tbsp wheatgerm oil
- 7 tsp rosewater
- 1 vitamin E capsule
- 2 drops each essential oils of rose, geranium, and black pepper

Melt the wax, cocoa butter, and oils in a bowl over a pan of boiling water, stirring continuously. Remove from the heat and mix in the rosewater, a few drops at a time, stirring until all the ingredients amalgamate. Prick the capsule and squeeze its contents into the cream as you mix in the essential oils. Spoon into a sterilized dark glass jar. Seal and refrigerate.

1 Pick up a little cream with the fingers of your right hand. Apply to the back of your left hand using smooth strokes from your fingertips up to your wrist.

2 Turn your left hand over. Cupping it with your right fingers, circle your palm with your right thumb. Apply more cream as needed as you stretch out the palm. Briefly press the center of your palm to promote relaxation.

3 Turn your left hand back over. Starting at your little finger, circle each knuckle with your right thumb. Slide down each of your fingers with your right thumb and forefinger. When you get to the fingertips, briefly squeeze to stimulate the brain and promote clear thinking.

4 Repeat steps 1-3 using your left hand to apply cream to your right. Interlink fingers and rub your palms together. Flex your fingers and shake your hands.

Moisturizing manicure

A weekly manicure is a self-affirming ritual that gives your self-esteem an invigorating boost every time you glance at your nails—visible proof that it's worth setting aside exclusive time for your hands. To increase this sense of invigoration, try some of the simple yet powerfully activating yoga exercises for the hands described below. Combine the manicures and pedicures in this chapter with any of the hair-conditioning treatments (*see pages 92-98*) for a feeling of complete restoration from head to toe. You will need a nail file, nail polish remover (optional), an orange stick, and lots of cotton balls.

Softening soak

- ½ lime or lemon
- 1 drop each essential oils of ylang ylang, neroli, and mandarin
- 1 tsp olive oil

To a bowl of warm, soapy water, add a squeeze of juice. Mix the essential oils into the olive oil. Pour into the water. Swish to disperse.

Energizing soak

- 1 tbsp freshly grated ginger root
- 2 drops each essential oils of orange and black pepper
- 1 tsp sesame oil

Heat the ginger in 1 cup of water and simmer, covered, for 10 minutes. Strain this infusion into a bowl of warm, soapy water. Mix the essential oils into the sesame oil. Pour into the ginger water. Swish to disperse.

Hand & wrist exercises

- Bring your palms together, elbows out, your thumbs lightly touching your sternum. Hold for at least 30 seconds. Close your eyes. Focus on slowing down and deepening your breathing. Try to repeat with your hands behind your back and your little fingers pressing into your spine.
- Stretch your arms forward, fingers straight and pointing upward, wrists extending forward, arms straight. Point your fingers down to the ground without moving your arms. Hold each position for at least 30 seconds. Feel the energy pumping forward and out through your wrists.
- Keeping your arms still, rotate your wrists in as wide a circle as possible, first out, then in. Repeat nine times in each direction.

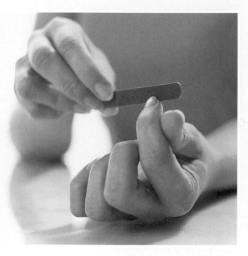

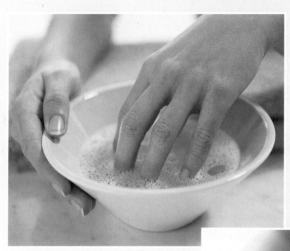

1 Remove old nail polish using an acetone-free remover. Sweep down from the cuticle to the tip of your nail without rubbing.

2 File your nails, working in from the outer edges using long, smooth strokes to create a rounded and oval shape.

3 Steep your hands for 2-3 minutes in either the Softening or Energizing Soak. Dry your hands and clean away any dirt residues from beneath the nails with an orange stick tipped with a cotton ball.

4 Stretch and wrap a clean cotton ball around the tip of an orange stick and gently push back the cuticles on each nail.

5 Moisturize with the Rich Hand Cream (*see page 81*) or your favorite hand cream product. Apply it to your nails last. Squeeze each one so the cream slips into the gap between the nail and the cuticle.

6 Once the cream has been absorbed, buff your nails with a chamois for a natural shine, or apply a formaldehyde-free nail varnish. Make one careful brushstroke down the middle of each nail and one on each side for a smooth, steady finish.

Footbath & massage

Bring tired feet back to life with a problem-specific footbath and foot massage. Soak and stretch your feet in one or two large bowls (or buckets), as you sip warming, detoxifying ginger tea. Gently massage your feet using pressure points and Tingling Foot Balm or Foot Massage Oil (*see pages 86-87*) and finish off with an application of Silky Dusting Powder.

Reviving sage & green tea footbath

- 1 tea bag, green tea
- 4 drops essential oil sage
- 6 sage leaves (optional)

Steep the tea bag in 1 cup of boiling water for 5 minutes. Remove it and pour the tea into a bowl of warm water. Add the essential oil and the sage leaves, if using. Soak your feet for 15 minutes. Ideal for tired, itchy, and sweaty feet.

Floral footbath

- 1 drop each essential oils of rose, jasmine, patchouli, and eucalyptus
- a handful dried lavender or seasonal flower petals

To a bowl of warm water, add the essential oils. Scatter in dried lavender or flower petals. Soak your feet for 15 minutes. Use anytime.

Ache-easing mustard footbath

- 1 tbsp mustard powder

To a bowl of very hot water, add the mustard powder. Stir to dissolve. Step in for 15 minutes. Wonderful for aching, painful feet.

Stimulating black pepper footbath

- 4 drops essential oil black pepper
- 4 drops essential oil peppermint

To a bowl of hot water, add the essential oil of black pepper. To a bowl of icy water, add the essential oil of peppermint. Keep your feet in the hot water for 5 minutes. Plunge them in the cold water for 2 minutes. Repeat 3 times. Perfect for overworked and swollen feet.

Silky dusting powder

- 8 tbsp cornstarch
- 3 drops each essential oils of rosemary and tea tree

Place the cornstarch in a wide jar with a lid. Add the essential oils. Shake. Use to give a satiny dusting to clean and dry feet.

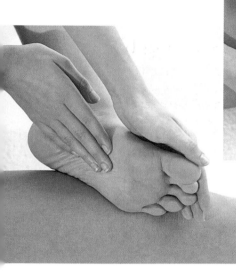

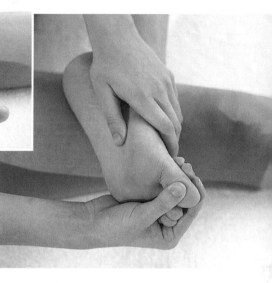

1 Rest your left foot above your right knee. Apply a little of the Tingling Foot Balm or Foot Massage Oil to one palm. Rub between both palms to warm it.

2 Sandwich your left foot between your hands. Roll your hands around your foot to spread the balm or oil. Rotate the knuckles of your right hand over the sole.

3 Walk your thumb up the center of the underside of your foot, then up either side of the sole, from your heel to the base of your toes. Creep your thumb down the outer edge from big toe to heel.

4 Support your toes with the fingers of your right hand. Firmly press the toes toward your left knee, then down toward the heel. Apply more oil or balm. Massage each toe, starting with your little toe and squeezing at the tip each time. When you reach the big toe, briefly apply pressure at its center with the tip of your thumb.

5 Circle your ankle and heel. With your forefinger and thumb, squeeze and release your Achilles tendon. Knead your way up your left calf, keeping your hand open and pressing with your thumb.

6 Stroke your right hand up your left foot from toe to knee. Repeat 1-6 on your right foot. Finally, rub a little balm or oil into your toenails.

Grounding pedicure

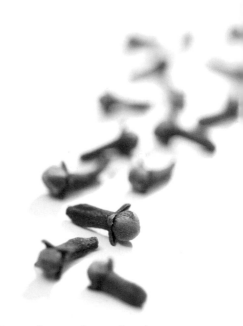

This once-a-week treatment removes dead skin cells as it softens and soothes the feet. The Softening Scrub is powerfully antibacterial and deodorizing relieving sore muscles and stimulating circulation. Very dry areas (like the heels) might benefit from the Exfoliating Fruit Mask. The Tingling Foot Balm, based on an Indonesian recipe, is particularly appealing to men and a powerfully aromatic tonic for perspiring feet . You will need a loofah, a nailbrush, a pumice stone, a nail file, an orange stick, cotton balls, plastic bags, and two warm towels.

Softening scrub

- 4 tbsp finely ground oatmeal
- 1 tsp ground ginger
- 1 tsp crushed cloves
- 1 tsp ground cinnamon
- 2 tbsp avocado oil
- 3 drops each essential oils of ginger and lemon
- 1 drop each essential oils of clove and cinnamon (optional)

Mix the oatmeal and spices with enough oil to make a dry paste. Stir in the essential oils. Rub over your feet and heels. Wipe away excess paste with a warm wet wash cloth. Splash your feet with warm water.

Exfoliating fruit mask

- 1 papaya
- 1 tbsp unpasteurized honey
- 1 tbsp sea salt
- 3 drops essential oil lemon

Scrape out the papaya flesh. Blend in a food processor with the honey and salt. Apply to your feet, focusing on very dry areas. Place a plastic bag over each foot. Cover with warm towels. Relax for 10 minutes. Discard the bags. Massage the mixture into your feet before showering them off with warm followed by cold water .

Tingling foot balm

- 15 g (½ oz) beeswax
- 100 ml (3⅓ oz) olive oil
- 5 drops each essential oils of coriander, lemon grass, and rosemary

Melt the wax and oil in a bowl over a pan of boiling water, stirring continuously. Remove from the heat and blend in the essential oils. Keep stirring until the cream cools. Spoon into a sterilized dark glass jar and seal. Refrigerate.

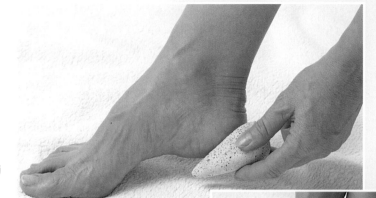

Foot massage oil

- 2 tsp sweet almond oil
- 1 tsp avocado oil
- 3 drops essential oil ginger
- 2 drops essential oil patchouli

Mix all the oils and apply to your feet, starting with the soles.

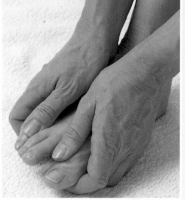

1 Remove old nail polish using an acetone-free remover. Sweep down from the cuticle to the tip of your nail.

2 Rub your feet with the loofah to stimulate circulation. Scrub your toenails with a nailbrush to get rid of any ingrained dirt. Use a pumice stone to remove layers of dry skin, especially around the heel and ball of your foot. Make long, sweeping movements in one direction.

3 Working from the outer edges in, file your nails with the nail file into a flat, square-edged shape.

4 Soak your feet, selecting one of the footbath recipes (*see page 84*). Pat your feet dry. Wrap a cotton ball around the orange stick and gently push back the cuticles on each toenail.

5 Apply the Softening Scrub or Exfoliating Fruit Mask. After rinsing, dry feet well. Take care to absorb all the moisture between your toes.

6 Moisturize your feet, one at a time, using the Tingling Foot Balm or Foot Massage Oil. Take care to work it between each toe. Lie on your back for 10 minutes with your buttocks gently pressed against the wall and legs raised. When the balm or oil has been absorbed, buff your nails with a chamois or apply a new coat of polish.

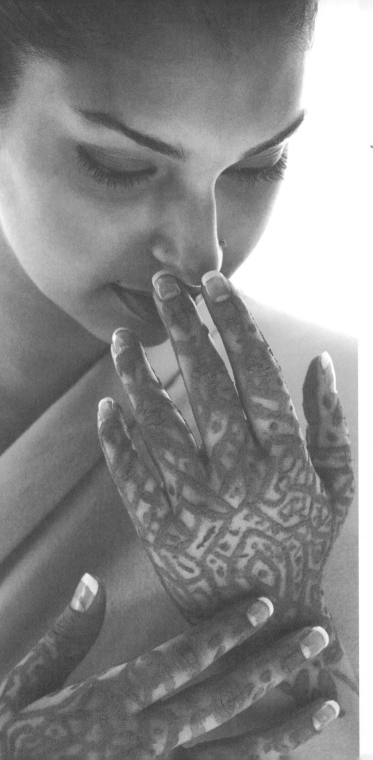

The art of mehndi

The art of *mehndi*—painting beautifully intricate, semi-permanent, henna designs to celebrate weddings or religious festivals—is synonymous with hands and feet in India, the Middle East, and Africa. Delicate tracings, paisley patterns, floral motifs, and geometric forms, some with ancient meanings, others with more modern inspiration, are selected from pattern books or suggested by *mehndi* artists. Modern *mehndi* patterns take their inspiration from Celtic, South American, or Taoist designs, as well as from Asian folklore and symbolism. When applying *mehndi* to yourself or a friend, you might like to try using pre-mixed cones, tubes with an attached nozzle, or do-it-yourself kits available from accessory and beauty care stores as well as Indian supermarkets. The designs last for up to three weeks.

Light mehndi mix

- 3 tbsp sifted henna powder

Make a paste by mixing the powder with warm water to a toothpaste-like consistency. Let it stand for 1 hour. Apply to skin and leave to dry for at least 2 hours. The paste stains skin for a few days.

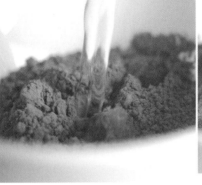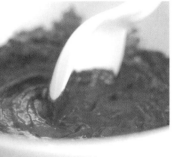

Deep mehndi mix

- 2 tea bags
- 3 tbsp sifted henna powder
- 1 tsp caster sugar
- 4-6 tbsp freshly squeezed lemon juice
- 2 drops each essential oils of tea tree, geranium, and cardamom

Pour 2 cups of boiling water over the 2 tea bags in a teapot. Steep for 5 minutes. Blend the powder and sugar with the juice into a stiff dough-type consistency. Moisten with cooled tea to a toothpaste-like thickness. Stir in the essential oils. Let it stand for 4 hours before use. Apply to skin. Leave to dry for at least 6 hours. The paste stains skin for up to 3 weeks.

Making a mehndi cone

Cut a 6 inch- (15 cm-) square from wax or greaseproof paper, polythene, or freezer bags. Roll it into a cone, leaving a tiny hole at the end. Tape up the seam. Fill the bag with either *mehndi* mix, twisting to close the top, or securing it with a freezer-bag tie.

1 Choose an appropriate design for your fingers or toes (like a stem-like motif) or your palm (like a rounded paisley shape).

2 If working on someone else, wear plastic gloves. Fill up a cone (*see above*) using the recipes given. Test the nozzle by squirting a little paste on a piece of paper first. Squeeze from one end and trace the pattern on your hand or foot. If you make a mistake, immediately wipe it away with a damp cloth.

3 When you have finished the design, keep your hand or foot away from water or anything that could smear it for at least 2 hours and preferably overnight.

4 Wait until it is dry before picking off any excess henna with your nails or a flat-bladed knife. Slip on cotton gloves before going to bed. Avoid using soap for at least 24 hours to preserve the coloring.

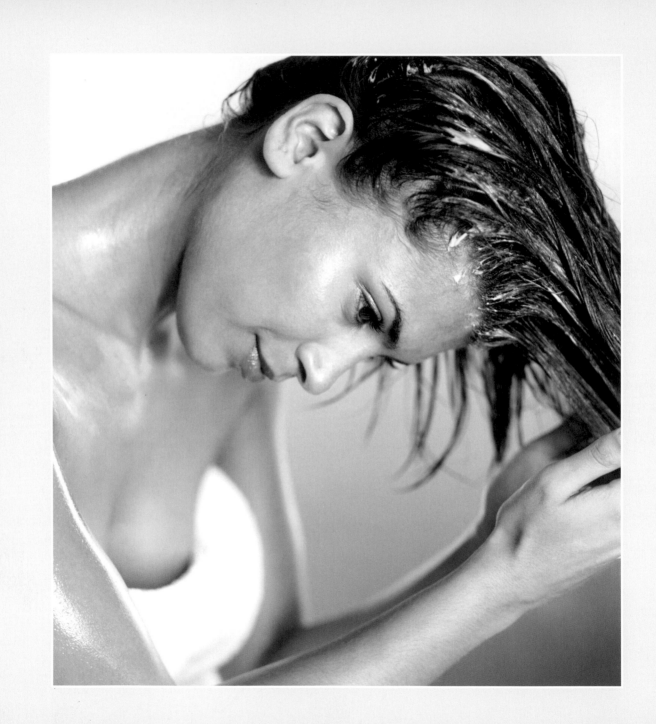

spice-infused haircare

Shiny, bouncy hair is a sign of good health and of the free-flowing movement of energy through the body. In Traditional Chinese Medicine, eating foods that support the lungs and the large intestine (the respective yin and yang organs linked to hair) is a key way to ensure energy moves into and around the body. For fabulous hair, include walnuts, black sesame seeds, seaweed, soya, ginger, coriander, cloves, and cinnamon in your diet. When choosing haircare products, opt for those made from nut oils, honey, healing plants, and sea extracts, and look for foaming agents other than the harsh chemical cleanser sodium lauryl sulphate.

Ayurvedic head massage

Bad hair days may be the result of poor circulation to your scalp. Increasing the flow of blood to the head helps nutrients reach the hair follicles, ensuring the growth of a healthy head of hair. The vital ingredients in head massage oils are also absorbed through the skin and add to the good condition of healthy hair. Massaging the scalp stimulates the entire nervous system, boosting your ability to concentrate and fighting stress. In Ayurvedic thought, applying oil to the head is believed to prevent hair loss and fight graying while strengthening the roots and leaving locks soft and glossy. Use this routine once a week or, if your hair is in need of drastic action, every night for a week, then weekly.

Blending scalp-massage oils

Add up to 10 drops in total of the essential oils to 1½ tbsp of carrier oil. Select a blend of your choice.

For dry, damaged, or colored hair: sandalwood, camomile, jasmine, and rosemary essential oils with coconut and sesame carrier oil; geranium and frankincense essential oils with macadamia carrier oil; lavender and camomile essential oils with sweet almond carrier oil.

For greasy hair: lemon, lime, juniper, and peppermint essential oils with sesame carrier oil.

For graying, mature, or thinning hair: camomile, lavender, and rose essential oils with avocado carrier oil; sandalwood essential oil with wheatgerm, sweet almond, and coconut carrier oils; juniper, rosemary, and black pepper essential oils with jojoba carrier oil.

Anti-dandruff scalp massage oil

- 2 tsp jojoba
- 2 tsp sweet almond oil
- 3 drops each essential oils of mandarin and lavender
- 2 drops each essential oils of juniper and rosemary

Mix the carrier oils together in a bottle. Drop in the essential oils. Shake well before use.

Dosha-specific massage oils

Warm the oil first by placing the bottle in a bowl of hot water.

Vatas: Use sesame or coconut oil.
Pittas: Choose from sunflower or coconut oil.
Kaphas: Select either mustard or sesame oil.

1 Mix the oil blend of your choice. Place a towel over your shoulders. Tap your fingertips over your scalp from between your eyebrows, up and over your forehead toward the crown of the head, and down to where your neck meets the base of your skull.

2 Pour a little oil into one palm. Rub it into the crown of your head. Applying a little more oil, rake your fingers down from the crown of your head to your ears, and then from your crown to the nape of your neck, combing your fingers through your hair.

3 Grab a handful of hair from either side of your head. Twist it clockwise, then anticlockwise. Bow your head. Apply more oil to the nape of your neck and spread it up over the top of your head to your forehead with your fingertips and back again.

4 Firmly rotate your left fingertips from your hairline above the left ear to the back of your head. Repeat with your right hand on the right side of your head. Twist and pull a handful of hair at the crown, the back of your head, and the nape of your neck.

5 Join your fingertips at the center of your forehead. Pull them outward to spread the oil. With your middle fingers, make anticlockwise circles at your hairline between the temples and your crown. Repeat this at the temples. With your index fingers, circle clockwise behind your ears, then gently press at the nape of your neck. Now make clockwise circles behind your earlobes.

6 Firmly rub your fingertips over the top of your scalp from your hairline to the back of your head and back again. Twist and pull the hair as in step 4.

7 Relax for 15-20 minutes before shampooing. If you're about to go to bed, leave the oil on overnight and cover your pillow with an old towel. Shampoo off the excess oil in the morning.

Natural
hair colorants

Spices and other aromatic plants have long been
used to tint or dye hair. In India, the leaves and
root of the sesame and the aloe vera plants are
used in hair-darkening decoctions. In Europe,
walnut, rosemary, and sage infusions bring
luster and dark tones to brown hair, while
camomile is the traditional friend of blondes.
Henna, with its unmistakable smell, is the
outstanding natural colorant from the world of
spices—when mixing your own powder, add a
teaspoon of ground nutmeg, cinnamon, or
allspice to mask the aroma without disrupting
the color. In the final stages of drying your hair,
hold it over a burning stick of sandalwood
incense and tousle with your fingers to ensure
the smoke scents every part of the hair before
finally styling.

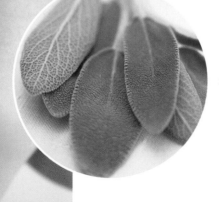

Sage makes a
pungent-scented
hair conditioner.

Magical henna

When first using henna, choose a ready-made recipe of herbs and natural colorants. Although normally associated with intense shiny reds, henna yields more subtle browns when mixed with coffee. A black-henna blend offers a chestnut glow, and an indigo mix gives a blue-black gloss. Follow packet instructions for mixing the henna. Do a strand test before applying henna to the whole head (especially with colored hair or graying hair). Apply to a finger-width strand of hair and note the time you leave it on. After drying, wait a couple of hours before treating the whole head as henna continues to color even after shampooing. It's always easier to brighten subtle colors than remove really intense tones. Wear rubber gloves, use old towels, and cover surfaces with newspapers. Wipe up any spills. Work on clean, dry hair. Divide it into small sections and apply the mixture with a brush from the roots down. For less intense tones, choose natural color washes made from tropical plants and spices. Use regularly for a few weeks to notice a difference.

Dark hair rinse

- 1 tea bag
- ½ lemon
- 4 drops essential oil sandalwood

Leave the bag to steep in 1 cup of boiling water. Combine with a good squeeze of juice and the oil. Use as a final rinse after shampooing to give a soft, dark complexity to black hair. Great for reducing hair loss.

Red-toned hair rinse

- 1 rosehip or hibiscus tea bag
- 1 tsp crushed cloves
- 2 drops each essential oils of orange and mandarin

Heat 1 cup of water in a pan. Add the tea bag and cloves. Cover and simmer for 20 minutes. When cool, strain, stir in the oils, and use as a rinse after shampooing.

Fair hair rinse

- 2-3 saffron strands
- 1 camomile tea bag
- 1 freshly squeezed lemon
- 4 drops essential oil lavender

Infuse the saffron in 1 cup of hot water. Pour 1 cup of hot water over the tea bag. Let both liquids steep for 20 minutes. Mix the lemon juice, saffron water, and camomile tea. Drop in the oil. Use as a final rinse for golden highlights.

Graying hair rinse

- 8 tbsp dried sage
- 4-5 sprigs fresh rosemary
- 3 drops essential oil ginger

Heat 2 cups of water in a pan. Add the sage and rosemary. Cover and simmer for 20 minutes. Allow to steep for 3 hours. Strain. Stir in the oil. Shampoo, then massage the liquid into any gray roots and leave on for 10 minutes. Rinse.

Conditioning secrets

Coconut is the wonder ingredient in many Eastern hair-luster treatments. The creamy texture of coconut oil and milk results from fatty acids resembling those of skin sebum, and is particularly suited to curly or dry hair. Coconut products also have protective antimicrobial properties to ward off harmful bacteria, yeast, and viruses. Traditional hair-conditioning treatments in the Maldives combine coconut oil with fenugreek, sandalwood, and cinnamon to boost blood circulation and stimulate the scalp. In Tahiti, coconut oil is infused with frangipani to produce softening and conditioning scented *monoi* oil. In Indonesia, women simply wash their hair in pure coconut milk.

Brittle & dry hair mask

- 2 tsp apricot kernel oil
- 1 tsp avocado oil
- 1 tsp jojoba
- 10 drops in total essential oils (choose from rose, ylang ylang, and jasmine)

Warm the oils in a bowl over a pan of boiling water, stirring well. Add the essential oils. Apply to hair from the roots combing through to the ends. Cover in plastic wrap and a warm towel. Relax for 15 minutes. Shampoo.

Anti-dandruff hair strengthener

- 1 tbsp sea salt
- 1 tsp ground licorice root
- 1 tsp dried, powdered mint
- 1 tbsp unpasteurized honey
- 1 drop each essential oils of peppermint and black pepper

Combine the salt and powdered herbs with enough honey to make a paste. Mix in the oils. Massage into your scalp for 10 minutes. Shower. Shampoo.

Conditioning avocado hair mud

- 2 tbsp avocado
- 2 tsp live natural yogurt
- 1 egg yolk (dry hair)
- 1 whole egg (oily hair)
- juice ½ lemon
- 2 drops each essential oils of sandalwood and rosemary

Blend all the fresh ingredients in a food processor. Mix in the essential oils. Massage into the scalp. Leave for 30 minutes. Rinse with cool water. Shampoo. Great for dry and weak hair.

Masala shiner

- 1 tsp each black peppercorns, coriander, and cumin seeds
- ¼ tsp each cloves, cardamom seeds, and ground cinnamon
- 1 tsp ground rose petals
- 2 tbsp coconut oil

Grind the spices with a pestle and mortar. Store them in a cool place. Warm 2 teaspoons of this mix with the ground rose petals in coconut oil for 15 minutes. Massage into dry hair. Cover with a plastic wrap and towel for 20 minutes. Shampoo.

Flower water splash

- 1 tsp rosewater or orange blossom water

Anoint your hands with a splash of the flower water. Sweep over your hair and circle your temples for a quick pick-me-up.

Maldivian scalp softener

- 1 tsp fenugreek seeds
- ½ crushed cinnamon stick
- 2 tbsp coconut oil
- 6 drops essential oil sandalwood

Warm the spices with the oil for 15 minutes in a pan. Strain. Mix in the essential oil. Massage into the scalp. Cover hair with plastic wrap and a warm towel. Leave on for 1-4 hours. Shampoo.

Perfumed hair oil

- 1½ tbsp coconut oil
- 10 drops in total essential oils (choose from rose, patchouli, bergamot, cedarwood, tangerine, and frankincense)

Stir the essential oils into the carrier oil. Dip your fingertips in the oil and massage into the hair before shampooing or use sparingly as an after-styling serum.

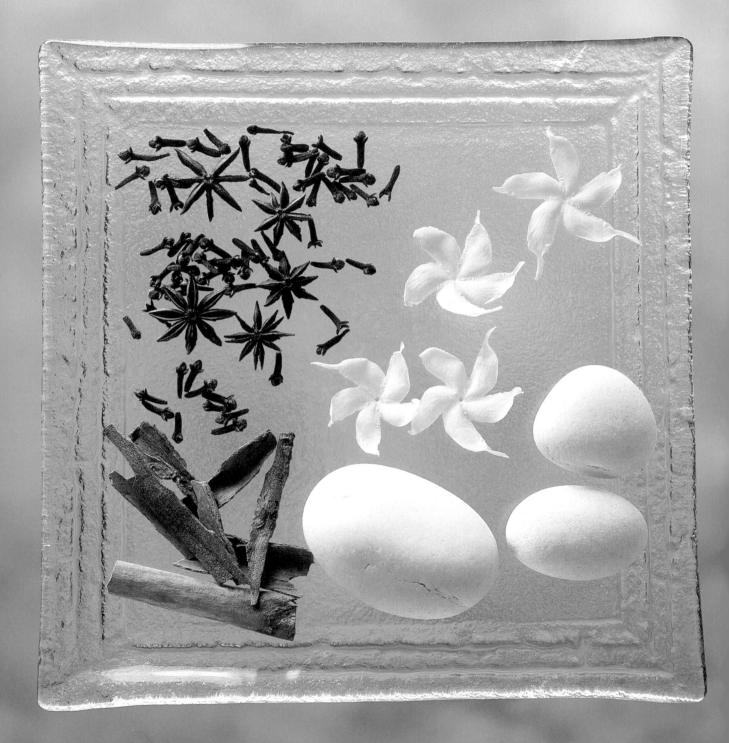

3

A glossary of spices

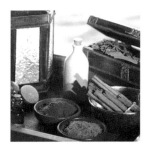

Spices are the aromatic dried parts of plants: the bark, roots, berries, buds, fruit, and seeds. They have been treasured for their curative effects since the earliest times. Most originate from Asia, others from the Americas and the Caribbean, a few from Mediterranean shores. Alongside spices, essential aromatic ingredients like honey, gram flour, nuts, grains, seeds, roots, resins, saps, fruit, and flowers help to make any beauty regime complete.

Cinnamomum zeylanicum

cinnamon

In oil-based scalp massages, tingling cinnamon strengthens and conditions hair as the massage strokes relax the mind. It makes a good addition to hair rinses, imparting a slight brown tone.

One of the oldest recorded aromatic plants, the cinnamon laurel is native to the forests of Sri Lanka and southern India. Once very rare, cinnamon came to be valued more highly than gold. It was traded aggressively from 1636 by the Dutch after they wrested Sri Lanka (then Ceylon) from the grasp of the Portuguese to become the most successful monopolizers of the cinnamon trade of their day.

The inner bark has been recognized by Indian, Chinese, and European medicinal traditions for its stimulating properties and its ability to reduce fevers, boost circulation, and lower blood pressure. Its antibacterial and antifungal properties make it effective as an inhalation for colds, while its antispasmodic action has been welcomed in treating digestive problems. Cinnamon is known to increase appetite levels; one of its constituents, cinnamaldehyde, is a proven sedative. In Chinese medicine, cinnamon is also valued for its pungent and sweet qualities and its effect on the "water" organs—the kidneys and the bladder.

For beautifying and medicinal purposes alike, cinnamon often is combined with ginger—in circulation-enhancing body scrubs (in Indonesia) and scalp-conditioning oils (in Malaysia). Cinnamon is used in incense and its oil is prized in perfumery.

When buying cinnamon, choose whole, smooth, tan-colored sticks (the paper-thin inner bark is hand-rolled into neat quills). Once ground, this spice tends to lose its woody yet sweetly sensuous aroma and warming intensity.

Caution: Avoid during pregnancy as it can be toxic in large doses. The essential oil is an irritant, so consult a qualified aromatherapist before using it in massage blends.

Coriandrum sativum

coriander

This fragrant perennial plant is native to western Asia and the Mediterranean and was cultivated by the ancient Babylonians as far back as the 8th century BCE. Roman merchants traded the herb far and wide and centurions carried the seed with them as they conquered lands to flavor their bread. By the 2nd century BCE, the fame of coriander had spread east to China, where it came to be appreciated as a digestive.

Medicinally, infusions of coriander calm the stomach and the intestines. The spice also acts to ease nervous tension. In India, coriander is ubiquitous in cooking and its medicinal effectiveness was praised in ancient Sanskrit texts, a tradition which still survives today when extracts of coriander are employed to cool the body and reduce fevers. In Indonesia, coriander seeds are a delicacy; in Thailand, the leaves and roots are favored.

Coriander is eaten throughout the world as a breath sweetener and a digestive, but in India, the whole plant is juiced for its astringent and cooling effect on the skin, particularly soothing for rashes and acne. Infusions are used to bathe the eyes. The essential oil of coriander makes a refreshing addition to any bath formula; it holds its own against heady Oriental scents in perfumery and is a major ingredient in incense mixes.

When buying coriander, choose seeds with a rich orangey, sweet yet peppery aroma, and grind them into powder form before use. Alternately, in the manner of Indian women, lightly dry roast the seeds before milling to bring out the flavor.

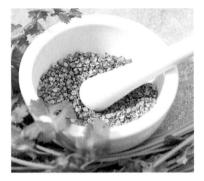

Coriander was a favorite beautifier of the ancient Egyptians, who regarded it as an aphrodisiac. Use the essential oil in sensual massage blends.

Crocus sativus

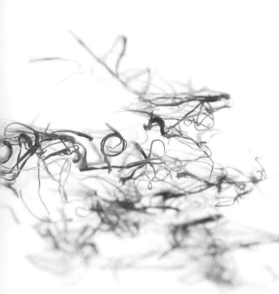

saffron

The three blood-red stigmas of this tiny violet crocus yield saffron, the world's costliest spice. Native to India and the eastern Mediterranean, historical records show it was cultivated extensively in medieval Europe as far west as Cornwall. Saffron was also honored in ancient Egypt, Greece, and Rome for its use as a brilliant gold dye, a sedative, and a perfume, as well as for its medicinal properties.

Its name derives from the Arabic *za'faran*, which means "yellow." Acclaimed as a powerful aphrodisiac and a sensual symbol of power and wealth, saffron was strewn over the routes of Roman emperors in golden carpets of the spice. Believed to promote compassion and devotion by Hindus and Buddhists, it is the dye of choice for monks' robes and is mixed with water into a paste to mark the forehead of devotees and anoint effigies of deities during Hindu religious festivals.

Saffron can help to ease period pains, bring on menstruation, relieve indigestion, and alleviate urinary disorders. In Indonesia, it is eaten during the dry season when sour, cooling ingredients are preferred to balance the body from within.

In beauty circles, saffron has a reputation for curing skin problems by softening and soothing. In India, a few saffron strands are infused in water, then added to the final rinse after shampooing to add russet lowlights to dark hair.

When buying saffron, choose fine, orange-red threads and expect to pay dearly for their bitter but heady muskiness. Avoid ready-ground saffron as it can be easily adulterated.

Caution: During pregnancy, avoid large doses.

Saffron is expensive to buy because it's so labor-intensive to produce: thousands of featherweight stigmas must be first handpicked, then dried, during a brief flowering period in the fall. For this reason, saffron has an aura of rarity that boosts its powerful sensuality when used sparingly as a water-soluble red dye in cosmetics, hair rinses, salves, and lotions.

Cuminum cyminum

cumin

This spice is native to Egypt's Nile Valley, where its healing properties were recognized over 5,000 years ago, and are still being used in herbal medicine today. This coriander-like plant with its clusters of white or pink flowers is described in the Old Testament as being threshed by rods, a practice still employed in the eastern Mediterranean before the seeds are left to dry in the sun.

Medicinally, cumin has been employed since ancient Egyptian times to stimulate the digestive system and relieve bloating by relaxing the intestinal muscles. In Ayurvedic medicine, it also is recommended as a remedy for indigestion and the roasted seeds arc infused in water to cure colds and fevers. In Indonesia, black cumin is considered warming and an antidote to stomach cramps, while the white variety is said to boost metabolism rates. Cumin is also reputed to combat insomnia. Its essential oil is well-regarded in perfumery and soap-making to balance highly floral scents such as lily of the valley.

When buying cumin, choose oval seeds with nine vertical ridges: their earthy, warming aroma is accompanied by a slight sharpness. Smaller black cumin seeds from Pakistan and Iran are finer and sweeter. To enhance their flavor, lightly toast the seeds in a dry pan until they change color before grinding them into a powder. Ready-ground cumin powder loses its pungency within a month or two.

Relaxing and rejuvenating, cumin helps combat insomnia, so reducing the telltale signs of lost sleep.

Curcuma longa

turmeric

Part of the ginger family, turmeric's Latin name, *curcuma*, derives from *kurkum* (Arabic) or *cuncuma* (Sanskrit). As these were also terms used for saffron, for centuries there was much confusion between the two spices. Traders exploited this by substituting turmeric—more readily grown and harvested—for costly saffron.

The ancient home of wild turmeric is southeast Asia, where it is treasured as one of the essential spices of *Jamu*—the Indonesian herbal healing and beauty tradition. Perhaps because its intense yellow color recalls the sun, turmeric took on sacred associations that still survive today. In India, the powder anoints and purifies Hindu brides and grooms before the wedding; when worn on the forehead during festival rituals, it brings divine energy to the wearer. Buddhist monks' robes are dyed with turmeric because it is more affordable than saffron and, in Indonesian temples, it is used to color ceremonial rice-cone offerings..

In India and China, these roots have long been renowned as a digestive tonic with the ability to stimulate the liver and gall bladder. In Java, where this spice is used in cooking and drunk as tea, gall bladder complaints are much less common than in the West. Turmeric maybe as effective as garlic in lowering cholesterol levels and even inhibits blood-clotting. Its yellow pigment is strongly antiviral and antibacterial. Turmeric also acts as an antioxidant, reducing the damaging effect of free radicals to skin cells, and as an anti-inflammatory agent to bring down swelling.

In terms of beautifying properties, turmeric boosts circulation, imparting a golden glow to darker-toned skin. Across Asia, it occurs in hair conditioners, purifying skin wraps, and face masks.

When buying turmeric, choose the fresh orange roots or the powder, which is just as effective.

For healing and beautifying alike, fresh turmeric root is grated or pounded into a powder, then mixed with a little water, milk, or oil before being applied to the skin. Once dry, its musky, resinous scent becomes more orangey and aromatic.

Cymbopogon citratus

lemon grass

With its distinctive, refreshing scent redolent of the delicate cuisines of Thailand and Vietnam, this tall, perennial grass is native to southern India and Sri Lanka, where it thrives in tropical climates. It is valued for its cleansing and relaxing properties.

Its constituent oils, citral (also found in lemon peel) and citronella, have long been shown to have a sedative effect on both mind and body, which accords with their long-term use in Eastern massage balms. In India, lemon grass is sipped in the form of tea to relax the muscles of the stomach and promote digestion, or it is applied externally as a diluted essential oil in a soothing abdominal massage. Prized as a cooling herb in both India and the Caribbean, lemon grass is infused in teas and applied locally as a poultice to induce perspiration and reduce fever. In Thailand, it is held in high regard for its pain-relieving, antiseptic, and antifungal properties.

The essential oil, which is steam-distilled from the lower shoots of the plant, is an essential aroma in Indian perfumery and is used to scent bath and hair oils. In Thai spas, the fresh stalks are pounded into a paste, then infused in boiling water, or chopped up with other ingredients to create masks, dry body rubs, and heated packs, renowned for their cleansing astringency. Used well-diluted in a massage oil, the essential oil of lemon grass offers a powerful relief to aching muscles, is a refreshing tonic for perspiring feet, and a vital ingredient of the traditional Indonesian coconut oil and musk mallow massage blend.

When buying lemon grass, select fresh stalks, breaking off a tiny piece to check the scent.

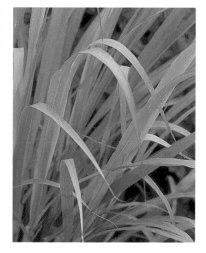

Lemon grass is used in bath, facial, and hair-rinse mixtures. It helps to regulate overactive oil glands and is effective for treating dry and oily skin, or dandruff.

Elettaria cardamomum

cardamom

This member of the ginger family is native to the rainforests of the Malabar Coast of India and Sri Lanka, but was being cultivated in the fabled hanging gardens of Babylon and traded in ancient Egypt.

As the world's third most valuable spice after saffron and vanilla, cardamom is costly to farm due to the amount of labor needed to hand-harvest the pods from the lily-like flower stems.

Medicinally, the constituent volatile oil in cardamom is a proven antispasmodic; in India, it has a long history of relieving indigestion and bloating, either applied in an abdominal massage-oil blend or drunk as an infusion. In China, cardamom is held to promote the flow of chi energy through the stomach and spleen. Cardamom infusions are taken both in India and Indonesia to combat coughs.

Roman gourmets recommended cardamom seeds to counter excessive eating. They are still proferred after an Indian meal and form part of the traditionally chewed betel-leaf digestive *paan*.

The ancient Egyptians regarded cardamom seed pods as a tooth whitener. They have been used to sweeten breath since those times because their constituent volatile oils slow the growth of bacteria which cause halitosis. In Indonesian herbal healing, cardamom is used to treat itchy skin. Its essential oil has been widely employed in perfumery for thousands of years

When buying cardamom, choose only the greenest and plumpest pods; those that are sharp-edged and difficult to break provide the best warmingly sweet but biting aroma. Crush the pods using a pestle and mortar to release the aromatic seeds.

Cardamom seeds are crushed for use in infusions or to extract the volatile oil. They make aromatic and warming digestive stimulants, especially effective against cramps and bloating.

Eugenia caryophyllata

clove

The closed, dried flower bud of this tropical species of myrtle tree was one of the earliest spices to be traded by Europeans from Indonesia's Maluku (Spice Islands). Stimulating to mind and body, cloves have enjoyed a long reputation as agents of sexual allure.

Medicinally, clove's constituent volatile oil contains eugenol, an ingredient with antibacterial, anesthetic, and antiseptic properties. In Indonesia, native Maluku medicine sees clove as a cure-all, where it is used to combat serious infections like malaria and tuberculosis. Another component, acetyl eugenol, is strongly antispasmodic and relieves indigestion, bloating, and coughs.

Clove oil is antispasmodic, effective in releasing stiff muscles through massage. In Bali, cloves are ground into the spicy, deep-heat, exfoliating *boreh* scrub treatment. They have an astringent effect on skin and calm acne and other dermal breakouts. Cloves are chewed to freshen breath and a few drops of the essential oil can be applied orally to relieve toothache. Indian women infuse cloves in tea and use it to tint gray hair strands. The essential oil of clove has been used in perfumery and soap manufacture since Roman times, and makes for an invigorating room fragrance as well—pomanders (oranges studded with cloves) have served as air fresheners in Europe since the Middle Ages.

When buying cloves, look for rich, red-brown, nail-shaped buds with intact, plump crowns and a woody, vanilla-tinged scent. Good-quality cloves emit small traces of oil when lightly pressed.

Caution: Do not use the essential oil during pregnancy. Consult a qualified aromatherapist before using in massage blends as the essential oil is a skin irritant.

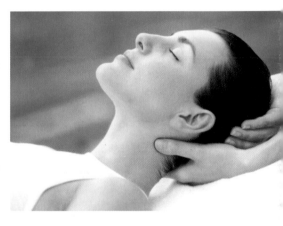

Cloves make a deliciously fragrant addition to cosmetic waters, lotions, and mouthwashes. When used in massage blends, the muscle-relaxing properties of the oil promote sleep. In potpourri sachets, cloves lift the spirit and the senses.

Foeniculum vulgare

fennel

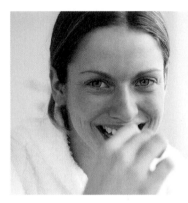

An infusion of fennel with eyebright makes a soothing eyewash and is reputed to have a strengthening effect on the eyes. Fennel seeds or the ground spice are also used in facial steams to open the pores.

The seeds of this perennial plant indigenous to the Mediterranean were once believed by medieval herbalists to be the panacea of all ills with the capacity to promote longevity and youthfulness.

Medicinally, this sweet spice is appreciated the world over for its ability to settle digestive complaints, as its constituent volatile oil has an antispasmodic effect on the muscles of the digestive system. In China, the warming energy of fennel is said to stimulate the flow of chi energy through the kidneys, bladder, and stomach. Gargling with an infusion of fennel is also recommended for sore throats. In India, roasted fennel seeds are believed to raise *agni* (digestive fire), and are chewed after meals to facilitate digestion.

For centuries, fennel has been used to brighten the eyes. Roman physicians recommended it for boosting eyesight and similar infusions are still in use in India to bathe sore eyes. The essential oil possesses detoxifying properties, effective in anti-cellulite massage oils. As part of facial massage blends, this oil helps revitalize dull and dry complexions.

When buying fennel, choose greenish-yellow, oval-shaped seeds for the best anise-like fragrance. Dry roast them before grinding to make the flavor more mellow.

Caution: Use sparingly as large amounts can be toxic. If you suffer from epilepsy, experience severe period pains, or are pregnant, do not use the essential oil.

Illicium verum

star anise

Native to southern China and Vietnam, this eight-pointed dried fruit of magnolia-species evegreen is considered to promote the flow of yang energy through the skin and the muscles, and is a key herb in detox diets to clear and purify skin. A defining spice in Chinese cuisine, star anise dominates five-spice powder, a blend of this spice and cassia, cinnamon, fennel, and cloves.

Medicinally, star anise is used in China to relieve rheumatism and back pain. Its muscle-relaxant and antibacterial properties also make this spice effective for treating digestive ailments.

This attractive fruit is well-respected in perfumery where it is used to scent soaps. In Japan, it is a traditional component of fine incense. In China, the eight points of the star fruit are chewed to freshen breath, and the spice is also brewed with scallions to create a tea that helps to help clear the spleen, kidneys, and liver.

When buying star anise, look for whole, hard, red-brown stars (the seeds are in the points). Crush them with a pestle and mortar to best appreciate the sweet, licorice-like aroma.

Associated with longevity—the tree bears fruit for up to 100 years—star anise may be used in massage blends to relax back muscles.

Lawsonia alba

henna

Synonymous with natural haircare, this evergreen shrub native to India, the Middle East, and North Africa, has prehistoric roots as a dye plant. Ancient Egyptian mummies were adorned with henna, perhaps because of its antibacterial and antifungal qualities, and wrapped up in henna-dyed cloth before burial. Henna is also traditionally entwined with the rich pageantry of Indian and Middle Eastern wedding ceremonies: most notably through the *mehndi* ritual, where women and girls gather around the bride to have hands and feet decorated with a variety of lacy latticework and floral henna designs on the day before the wedding.

Medicinally, henna leaves are infused to make a soothing gargle for sore throats and to treat serious intestinal complaints such as dysentery. The leaves have an astringent effect and screen ultraviolet light. When applied as a paste, henna alleviates acne and other skin complaints. Henna both prevents hemorrhaging and is used by Indian women to bring on menstruation.

The key beautifying use of henna is to bring semi-permanent color and lustrous gloss to dull, lifeless hair. Different species of the plant, or mixes of henna with other herbs (such as indigo), offer a whole selection of hues, from ebony and mahogany, to copper tones and the signature deep-red. The strong-scented henna leaves have a long history of use in perfumery.

When buying henna, select the ready-ground, powdered khaki-green leaves. Mix with hot water into a sticky consistency, and apply to hair. Ready-mix tubes of henna paste for *mehndi* are widely available from some Asian stores and accessory and beauty care stores.

The act of adorning hands and feet with intricate henna patterns is traditional to weddings and religious feast days in India, Asia, Africa, and the Middle East. Since the 1990s, it has also found favor in the West as a form of temporary tattoo.

Myristica fragrans

nutmeg and mace

These spices derive from the fruit of the nutmeg tree native to the Banda Islands in Maluku (the Spice Islands), Indonesia. Nutmeg is the seed inside the hard kernel of this apricot-like fruit; mace is the lacy filigree covering it. Valued in the West since Roman times, nutmeg was strewn on streets before an emperor's coronation. In India and Indonesia, nutmeg and mace are libido-boosters; in the provinces of Kalimantan, in Borneo, the pink-red sap of the tree is known as *pendarah* (blood), and thought to be magically potent. The constituent ingredient myristicin, far greater in mace than in nutmeg, is highly toxic (even in small quantities) and is a euphoria-inducing hallucinogen similar to mescaline.

Medicinally, nutmeg and mace share various properties. Valued in Indian, Chinese, and Arabic medicine, nutmeg eases intestinal and stomach disorders thanks to its stimulating and anesthetizing effect on the digestive system. As an ointment, it soothes rheumatism. In the native herbalist tradition of Kalimantan, mace is thought to cure headaches, and Ayurvedic medicine prescribes nutmeg, the most sedative of all the spices, for insomnia.

In India, a little nutmeg powder mixed with water into a paste is used to treat skin problems like eczema. The essential oil stimulates and warms the skin, while a little nutmeg oil combined with lemon grass makes a stimulating Balinese massage blend.

When buying nutmeg, choose whole nuts that yield a little oil when lightly pressed. Grate them just before use. Enjoy the nutty fragrance, slightly sweeter for nutmeg than for mace. Yellow-red powdered mace preserves its aroma best of all.

Caution: Do not use during pregnancy.

Powdered nutmeg may be combined with a variety of other spices such as black pepper, cardamom, and clove in a *masala*-inspired body rub.

Nigella sativa

nigella

Long-respected in many cultures for their curative and restorative powers, nigella seeds are strongly antiseptic.

Nigella seeds come from a relative of the feathery love-in-a-mist plant and are native to western Asia and the Mediterranean.

Medicinally, nigella eases abdominal pain, bloating, and indigestion. It relieves headaches, acts as a diuretic, and helps to boost a nursing mother's milk supply.

For beautifying, mix the seeds with a little water. Apply to the skin to help prevent and reduce spots, pimples, and blackheads.

When buying nigella, choose five-pointed, oregano-scented, matt-black seeds (not be confused with black cumin). Dry roast and mill in a coffee grinder to bring out the nutty, peppery aroma.

Papaver somniferum

poppy

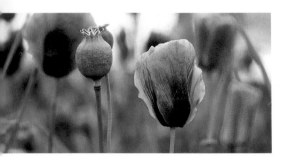

The alkaloids in opium poppy seeds are analgesics and, in cultures around the world, the spice is considered to be an energy booster.

These seeds derive from the opium poppy of western Asia, one of the oldest plants in continuous cultivation. Poppy seeds do not share the analgesic properties derived from the latex exuded by their fresh seed capsules, which is used to make narcotics.

Medicinally, poppy seeds are used antispasmodically to ease stomach and intestinal disorders from cramping to indigestion.

Poppy seeds are astringent and add texture to emollient preparations like skin-polishing masks and body scrubs.

When buying poppy seeds, select whole, blue-gray ones and dry roast them before milling in a coffee grinder. In India, white seeds are the preferred variety. Both types have a nutty sweetness.

allspice

Pimenta officinalis

Jamaica pepper, or allspice, is the dried unripened fruit of a long-lived species of myrtle. Its perfumed aroma is a complex mix of spices, including nutmeg, cloves, cinnamon, and pepper. It is one of only a few New World spices in the international spice box. After being introduced to Europe by Christopher Columbus, allspice became a staple of international trade between the 17th and 19th centuries. Its preservative qualities were exploited by the Mayan Indians for embalming.

Medicinally, allspice and its essential oil are effective in easing digestive complaints and have stimulant and antiseptic properties.

A traditional part of room-fragrancing potpourri, allspice is a respected ingredient in men's perfumery, where its spicy aroma holds its own alongside other rich scents.

When buying allspice, choose whole, reddish-brown berries from Jamaica for the best quality.

Caution: Do not use the essential oil during pregnancy.

Generally used in powder form, allspice is found in hair rinses because of its color-inducing properties and pleasantly spicy scent; in perfumes and cologne; and as an astringent or freshener in bath herbs, ointments, and creams.

Pimpinella anisum

anise

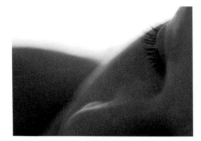

Cosmetically, anise is used in facial steams to open up pores. Drunk before going to bed, aniseed tea helps your skin reap the full benefits of a good night's sleep.

The seeds of this annual plant native to the eastern Mediterranean and the Middle East have been used to relax and revive for over 4,000 years. Anise, or aniseed, was served in Roman times as a digestive, and is widely available in India as sugar-coated comfits eaten to help digestion after a heavy meal.

Ancient Egyptian and Roman physicians, like modern Ayurvedic practitioners, prescribed chewing anise seeds to settle digestive disorders and relieve trapped wind, bloating, and other discomforts. The antispasmodic properties of aniseed are also used to treat painful periods, asthma, and respiratory ailments. Anise is noted for its diuretic qualities, as a fungicide, and to boost a nursing mother's milk supply.

For beautifully rested skin the next day, infuse anise seeds in hot water and drink as a tea before going to sleep. Anise seeds are chewed for fresh breath the world over, while in India, an infusion of anise water is used as eau de cologne.

When buying anise, hand-pick whole, oval seeds for the freshest zesty fragrance and lightly dry roast them before use.

Caution: Do not use during pregnancy.

Piper nigrum

black pepper

Literally worth its weight in gold, black pepper derives its name from *pippali,* the Sanskrit word for "berry." From prehistory, pepper was traded west of its native Malabar Coast in southwest India by Arab traders, who closely guarded the secret of its origins. The ancient Greeks knew of black pepper by the 4th century BCE, and the Romans used it as a war tribute and a means of imposing tax. Lust for pepper, the most sought-after spice in medieval Europe, led Europeans to seek sea routes to the East.

Medicinally, pepper has been valued as a stimulant for the digestive system and for its antiseptic and antibacterial action (in East Africa, eating black pepper is said to repel mosquitoes). Its essential oil acts on the circulation by dilating blood vessels, which explains its long use in massage oil blends to reduce muscular aches (especially back pain), rheumatism, and fever.

Crushed black peppercorns, highly valued for their protein content and mineral mix, are used in warming body scrubs (particularly enjoyed by men) to heat muscles and increase circulation. Black-pepper Ayurvedic preparations are believed to burn up *ama* (toxins) and combat acne. In perfumery, this spice mixes well with other heady Oriental-style scents.

When buying black pepper, select large, whole peppercorns (the unripe berries of this tropical vine), which have been fermented briefly before being sun-dried. They contain more of the volatile oil than white peppercorns which are the dried berries with the outer skin removed. Freshly grind the corns to best savor their sharp pungency and earthy aroma.

Caution: Avoid the essential oil if taking homeopathic remedies.

Spas and natural skincare companies are increasingly exploiting the naturally powerful, heat-penetrating properties of black pepper in beauty preparations, recipes, products, and treatments.

Punica granatum

pomegranate

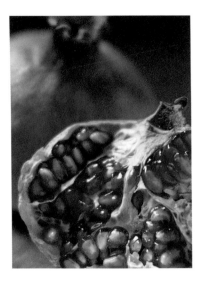

Pomegranate juice and the pulp-like tissue of the crimson grains make an excellent external astringent for oily skin and a highly stimulating hair oil for glossy, shiny tresses.

The seeds of this strange-looking fruit native to southwest Asia form the spice. The sweet-sour, jewel-colored fruit, and its brilliant scarlet-flowered tree, are the stuff of legend, celebrated as a symbol of abundance, prosperity, and fertility in Hindu, Christian, and Turkish lore. The pomegranate is said to have been the original "apple" of the Tree of Knowledge in the Garden of Eden, while in Islamic tales, the Prophet Mohammed recommends eating this fruit to purge oneself of envy and hatred.

Medicinally, the ability of pomegranate rind and bark to rid the body of tapeworm has been extolled since ancient Egyptian times, a cure also common in ancient Rome and India. In modern-day Spain, people drink pomegranate juice to settle an upset stomach. In India, it is believed to cleanse the blood by encouraging the production of new red blood cells.

Pomegranate seeds form part of an Indian woman's traditional beauty kit. Their highly astringent, fleshy juice with its valuable antioxidant fruit acids is applied as a mask to close pores and treat excessively oily skin.

Buy either fresh pomegranate fruit, or look for the dried seeds or powder of *anardana* (a sour variety of the fruit). In Middle Eastern stores, look for pomegranate syrup. To use, simply scoop out the juicy seeds fresh from the fruit.

Caution: Do not use the rind or bark unless prescribed by a qualified herbalist.

sandalwood

Native to eastern India, sandalwood has been considered sacred for centuries. Thought to promote meditation and deepen spirituality, the wood from this evergreen tree is used to carve scented prayer beads and forms part of the paste which makes the *tilak* marks on the forehead of Hindu devotees.

Medicinally, the wood from the heart of this tree has been recognized as a remedy for chest and abdominal pains in China. In Ayurvedic medicine, its antiseptic essential oil (extracted from 50-year-old trees) eases skin conditions and genito-urinary problems such as cystitis. Its cooling effect is valued in treatments for fever and inflammation.

Astringent sandalwood heals and tones dehydrated or sensitive skin. In India, the powder is mixed with turmeric and milk for a cooling face or body mask. Balinese women use the essential oil of sandalwood in conditioners for dry, damaged hair, and Indian women scent their hair over sandalwood-smoking incense burners. To discourage the growth of facial hair, Ayurvedic practitioners advise using a paste of sandalwood and clay left on overnight twice a week. After shaving, a few drops of sandalwood oil in a carrier oil help to soothe inflamed skin. Ayurveda considers sandalwood to be the best essential oil for calming the mind and rejuvenating the nerves: burn it in a vaporizer during treatments to relax and sedate.

When buying sandalwood, look for the best-quality variety which always comes from Mysore and is goverment-controlled. This type of sandalwood might not look different, but it has a particularly intense balsamic, syrupy, wood-like scent.

Synonymous with beauty products and perfume materials generally, sandalwood also has medicinal uses: applied externally to wounds, it acts as a disinfectant; added to bath mixtures in the form of chips, it works as an antiseptic.

Sesamum indicum

sesame

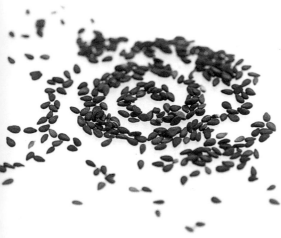

Sesame oil is externally effective as a soothing emollient in massage and bath oils, body lotions, wraps, salves, and creams. An excellent massage base, it calms and nourishes skin.

Although native to Africa and possibly India, sesame seeds arrived in China about 5,000 years ago, where the oil from the black variety was burnt to make ink and used as a staple ingredient in cooking. These seeds were believed to bring good fortune by African slaves. In parts of southern India, they are considered auspicious, capable of increasing *ojas* (life sap), and bringing about spiritual growth. Southern Indian brides are playfully adorned with garlands and bangles of candied seeds.

In Africa and India, the seeds are ingested to ease stomach disorders. In China, they serve as a tonic to rebalance the liver and kidneys. In India, where the black variety is considered most healing, such seeds are thought to be regenerative and aphrodisiac.

Crush the sesame seeds in a warming body wrap to ease aching muscles and joints, or use them as the base for a traditional Thai body scrub (with honey and mint). Sesame oil makes the perfect carrier for massage oils. Ayurveda teaches that it penetrates the skin deeply, nourishing and detoxifying it at the deepest level and also advises rubbing sesame seeds into body and scalp for winter warmth. Indian women wash a decoction of sesame leaves and roots into the hair to combat graying, while in China, black sesame seeds are both a scalp-stimulating, anti-graying hair treatment, as well as an antidote for dry skin.

When buying sesame, look for creamy, glossy seeds and bear in mind that the black variety have the strongest flavor. Toast them lightly to release their nutty aroma. For mixing body masks, use bottled Middle Eastern *tahina* paste (made from finely ground seeds). For massage purposes, choose light-colored sesame oil over its darker-hued Chinese or Japanese equivalent, which is pressed from toasted seeds.

Tamarindus indica

tamarind

This decorative tree, native to Madagascar, is more commonly known as the "Indian date," perhaps because the pulp and seeds within its brittle, crescent-shaped pods have been used in India as a souring and cooling agent for centuries. The seeds have holy associations and are first boiled, then mixed into a paste to create the colors traditionally used in sacred paintings—white, yellow, black, green-brown, red, gold, and silver.

Tamarind is used in herbal medicine to cleanse the digestive system and serve as a warm gargle to soothe sore throats. Ayurvedic practitioners recommend the ripe tamarind fruit for bowel problems and to strengthen digestion, and use poultices of its leaves to treat inflamed joints. In China and Indonesia, tamarind is appreciated as a digestive tonic and for its cooling properties. Similarly, in the Middle East and the Caribbean, it is enjoyed as a cooling summer drink.

In Indonesia, tamarind oil is frequently used in beauty treatments. The high vitamin content of its young leaves is nourishing when applied to inflamed and irritated skin. The pulp is an active ingredient in astringent face masks for oily skin. In Thai spas, tamarind water adds moisture to dry body wraps.

When buying tamarind, purchase pressed blocks—a sticky, dried mass of pods and pulp. Break off a little and soak it in warm water until pulpy, then squeeze its fibrous mass between your fingers to extract the thick brown juice. Strain before use. Alternately, look for jars of concentrate with a sour yet fruity flavor in Asian and Caribbean grocers.

Caution: Do not use during pregnancy.

Cooling tamarind water and its pithy pulp impart an astringent tartness and add moisture to face masks, tonics, and detoxifying body wraps.

Vanilla planifolia

vanilla

The dried seed pod of an orchid that flowers for a single day, vanilla is nurtured to maturity for a period of up to nine months. Its name derives from the Spanish *vainilla*, meaning "little pod." Native to Mexico, vanilla is sacred to the Totonaca people of the Gulf Coast, who have cultivated it since Mesoamerican times. Its use spread to Europe after Spanish conquistador Hernan Cortés reached Mexico in 1520, and was offered a rich, local Mayan concoction of chocolate, vanilla, and spices. The Aztecs considered vanilla to be an aphrodisiac.

Medicinally, the Mexican Totonaca people blended this spice with other native plants to treat respiratory ailments and digestive problems. They also used it to fragrance their homes and modern research has shown that the scent of vanilla reduces anxiety and induces relaxation. Skin patches containing vanilla may even reduce cravings for sweet foods.

For beautifying, steep vanilla pods in hot water for a rich, exotic, floral bath. Let the pods dry afterward so they can be used over and over. Alternately, scent the final rinse water with the pods after conditioning your hair. In the Maldives, vanilla pods are infused in coconut milk to create a pampering body lotion—a practice that resembles that of the Totonaca, the first people to apply vanilla oil to skin for a glossy sheen. Vanilla is also highly prized as a concentrate in perfumery.

When buying vanilla, either choose pods from Réunion or Madagascar, which are superior and coated in vanillin, a white crystal frosting, or purchase real vanilla essence. Avoid any artificial vanilla flavoring and do not skimp on the cost.

Vanilla beans are used in dry potpourris, drunk as an aphrodisiac in hot chocolate, and infused in body massage oils. Harvesting vanilla requires blanching, sweating, and curing the pods to ensure they retain their suppleness once dried.

Zingiber officinale Alpinia officinarum

ginger and galangal

Hailed as the panacea among spices, ginger is considered a wonder drug in Asian herbal healing traditions. Galangal, another member of the ginger family, native to China and southeast Asia, shares similar healing qualities.

Ginger is particularly renowned for treating digestive ailments from nausea to food poisoning. It can be drunk as a tea, juice, or infusion, chewed in slices, or blended into a massage oil. The stimulating action of ginger comes from zingiberene, its active volatile oil, and ginerol, another constituent ingredient. Ginger and galangal boost circulation, fight inflammation, and ease muscular and arthritic discomfort. Powerfully antibacterial, antifungal, and antiseptic, both spices promote perspiration, break fevers, and soothe the symptoms of colds and flu.

When applied to broken or irritated skin, pounded ginger promotes healing. Galangal is used in a similar way, ground with a variety of indigenous natural ingredients (such as pepper), to soothe skin. When diluted in carrier oils (such as jojoba) in massage blends, the essential oil is an excellent detoxifier. Applied as a warm compress to skin, ginger is considered regenerative for both mind and body; a paste of ginger, cinnamon, and cloves or aloe vera applied to the head before sleep is a good headache cure.

When buying ginger or galangal, select firm, shiny, fresh roots, and check whether they ooze fragrant juice. Avoid woody or stringy ones. Peel and grate finely before use. Jamaican ginger has a delicate piquancy. Greater galangal has a more sour, peppery tang, and Lesser galangal reveals a hint of cardamom.

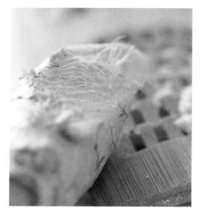

In Indonesia, ginger is a key ingredient in herbal weight-loss products. It is considered to be an extremely effective body toner. Used in body wraps, ginger can help new mothers get their shape back after childbirth in just six weeks.

other essential aromatics

From country to country and across world traditions, spices have been blended with the natural harvest of earth, ocean, and dairy to create rebalancing beauty preparations for all skin types.

nuts, beans, seeds, & grains

soya

Considered the ultimate beauty food in Japan, soya is rich in phytoestrogens and vitamin E. It promotes a youthful complexion and restores vitality to tired-looking skin. Ayurvedic medicine recommends using it as tofu, its most digestible form.

mustard

Mustard seeds have stimulant, diuretic, and analgesic properties. Mustard oil is used in warming winter-scalp massages in India for strong, lustrous hair. The recommended detox massage oil for kapha types
(see pages 14-15).

candlenut

The oil adds shine and gloss to hair, prevents graying, and.is a body moisturizer and exfoliator.

almond

Packed with protein and vitamins, almond can be a revitalizing skin soother. Ground almond paste is applied as a daily face mask, followed by almond milk as a cleanser. Choose sweet almond oil as a light, soothing base for massage blends. The recommended facial oil for kapha types *(see pages 14-15)*.

coconut

Coconut husks make a natural pumice for rough feet. Coconut milk is mixed into body lotions to nourish the skin and is also used in shampoos. Warmed coconut oil makes a scented, conditioning hair treatment. It is recommended for moisturizing chapped lips and treating skin blemishes. The essential detoxifying massage and facial oil for pitta types *(see pages 14-15)*.

chickpeas & gram flour

The source of gram flour or *besan*, chickpeas are great antioxidants that stimulate the immune system and provide a base for skin masks and rubs.

rice

Believed to contain the energy of yin and yang. In powder form, the base for Indonesian body scrubs. Mix rice powder with rose water (for normal skin), with milk (for dry skin), or tamarind (for oily skin). Use rice water for a rich face lotion.

roots & saps

ginseng

The key tonic herb in Chinese medicine, ginseng calms the spirit, brightens the eyes, opens the heart, tones the body, and promotes longevity. Its root brings a fresh, abundant flow of chi, which enhances vitality, increases resistance to stress, and nurtures restorative sleep. It strengthens hair roots and restores the skin's natural pH. **Caution:** Do not take during pregnancy or for more than six weeks as the ginseng loses its effectiveness and may be harmful. Do not mix with caffeine. Avoid large doses.

frankincense

Used in facial steams and inhalations, this scent boosts meditation and deepens breathing. Its essential oil is anti-inflammatory and antiseptic, effective for treating chapped skin and wrinkles.

fruit

papaya

Its seeds and skin are full of revitalizing vitamins A, C, and the active enzyme papain. A powerful digestive and antioxidant, papaya is a cooling yin food and a natural source of alphahydroxy acid, prized for gentle exfoliation. Ripe puréed papaya flesh can be applied as a body mask or around the eyes to soften wrinkles. Its leaves are used to dress wounds. Scoop out the inner skin and massage into the face as an exfoliating rub.

mango

A highly effective astringent face mask ingredient.

lime

The vitamin C-rich juice is highly astringent and draws out toxins. It also moistens dry ingredients in body masks and scalp stimulants.

avocado

Mash and apply the pulp as a soothing face mask, or as a cooling, growth-promoting hair conditioner. Rinse off with cold water. Avocado oil is a rich emollient and a plentiful source of vitamins A, B_1, B_2, B_6, C, and E, protein, and monounsaturated fats. The recommended facial oil for vata types *(see pages 14-15)*.

banana

This plant's high potassium levels and high vitamin content (A, B_6, E, and F) make it a soothing, rehydrating mask for dry or mature skin and a gentle hair growth stimulant.

from earth & sea

salt

French thalassotherapy centers and Eastern spa resorts use the healing properties of unrefined crystals harvested from the sea in various beauty treatments to draw out toxins and rid the skin of layers of dead cells. White rock salt (the Indian variety is dark-colored) is mined from underground water sources and the best sea salt is evaporated from sea water by the wind and the sun. Look for Breton unrefined *sel aux algues* sea salt crystals with flecks of seaweed or Japanese salt blended with sesame.

seaweed

From dark Japanese *kombu* to curly *hijiki*, from green *wakame* to dried *nori* sheets, seaweed shares the chemical make up of human plasma, and is a rich source of vitamin B_{12}, potassium, calcium, and iron. Strongly antioxidant, it helps to stimulate the immune system.

Thalassotherapy recommends exercise in sea water with seaweed wraps. Japanese *arame* has a detoxifying effect when massaged into areas that are prone to cellulite.
Caution: Do not use if pregnant or while breastfeeding as the detoxifying effect may be too intense.

clay

In deep-cleansing face masks and cellulite treatments, clays tighten the skin to draw blood up to the surface and absorb any impurities. Thai "white mud" (*din so porng*) prevents sun damage to the skin, acts as a natural antiperspirant, and can be mixed with turmeric, oils, herbs, and milk to create purifying body masks.

oils & balms

milk, cream, & natural yogurt

Thought to be especially nourishing for the complexion, these substances are used to moisten the drier ingredients of masks and wraps. Natural yogurt makes for a softening and cooling face mask.

honey

Thought to encourage the free flow of chi, raw honey is an ancient wonder food for skin. Packed with vitamins B, C, and E, the ability to destroy free radicals, and humectant properties, honey is also a powerful wound cleanser and healer. Choose cold-processed New Zealand honey because it is made from the nectar of the amazingly healing manuka tree, whose essential oil is 33 times more effective in destroying skin bacteria than tea tree oil.

aloe vera

The thick, sticky leaf sap accelerates the healing of wounds, soothes irritated skin, and reduces blemishes. The clear gel is used in hair treatments to stimulate growth and develop color.

flowers

hibiscus

Its red petals can be boiled to make a hair colorant that adds luster and promotes growth. When mashed up with water, the leaves create an effective shampoo.

jasmine

The essential oil is used in massage blends, scrubs, and lotions for its calming, sedative effect on the nervous system. The oil is especially softening for dry, sensitive skin. **Caution:** Do not use the essential oil during pregnancy.

rose

Gentle face masks are made from rose petals and astringent rosewater is a valued skin toner. The essential oil gently restores mature or inflamed skin, can reduce the appearance of thread veins, and guards against wrinkles. Choose rose attar over the cheaper, less pure absolute.

ylang ylang

This heady essential oil is said to be an aphrodisiac and is used in bath oil treatments. **Caution:** Dilute the essential oil well (*see page 61*).

patchouli

An effective skin soother, its antibacterial properties improve skin tone and clear up blemishes. Great for mature skin. A good addition to hair oils for dry scalps. The essential oil is an aphrodisiac and an antidepressant.

Index
a-b

Carroll & Brown Limited would like to thank:

Editorial Assistant: Stuart Moorhouse

Design Assistant: Jim Cheatle

Photography Assistant: David Yems

Production Director: Karol Davies

Production Controller: Nigel Reed

IT Manager: Paul Stradling

Picture Researcher: Sandra Schneider

Indexer: Madeline Weston

Susannah Marriott would like to thank everyone at Carroll and Brown, especially Anna Amari-Parker for being ever patient and attentive to detail. Thanks also to Roshan and Salima Hirani and to the following for kindly supplying recipes, images, and information: Julia Gajcak and Luisa Anderson at The Island Spa, Four Seasons Resort Maldives, Kuda Huraa, North Male Atoll (www.fourseasons.com); Izan Yusuff at Spa Village, Pangkor Laut Resort, Pangkor Laut Island, Malaysia (www.ytlhotels.com); Sisadhi Christopher Reuben at The Oriental, Bangkok, Thailand and Nina Colls and Lindsey Hughes at Mandarin Oriental Hyde Park, London, United Kingdom (www.mandarin-oriental.com); Anez Taufik at The Source, Begawan Giri Estate, Payangan, Ubud, Bali, Indonesia (www.begawan.com); Sarah Noble and Bacall Associates for Chiva-Som, Hua Hin, Thailand (www.chivasom.com).

Sourcing beauty care ingredients

Most of the ingredients used in the recipes in this book—honey, flour of different types, yogurt, nuts, and fruit—are available from larger supermarkets or health food stores. For spices and herbs, try Indian, Pakistani, Middle Eastern, Thai, and Vietnamese shops as they offer the best selection of spices: often fresher and of better value than those on the supermarket shelves. The shopkeepers may also be willing to share beauty care knowledge from their own cultural backgrounds.

Look for essential oils in health and natural beauty stores. Choose organic where possible. For salts, seaweed, clay, and ginseng, pay a visit to your local health food store. If they don't stock what you're after, a small, independent shop may order it for you. For organic products, visit organic supermarkets or try farmer's markets and farm shops for local specialities like honey or dairy produce.

The following are superb spa product ranges, some of which avoid using animal or GM ingredients: E'spa, Elemis, Aveda, Sundari, Origins, Dr Hauschka, Jurlique, Thalgo, REN, Living Nature, Korres, and Aesop.

Picture Credits

Andrew Lawson p. 105; **Camera Press/Jahrezeiten-Verlag** p. 38, p. 47; **Camera Press/Mise en Image** p. 69; **Chiva-Som International Health Resort, Hua Hin, Thailand** p. 17, p. 67, p. 107; **Corbis/Paul Anthony** p. 88; **David Murray** p. 116; **Four Seasons Resort Maldives, Kuda Huraa, The Island Spa** p. 1, p. 2, p. 8, p. 9, p. 11, p. 29, p. 78, p. 98, p. 99; **Getty Images** p. 75 (r), p. 80, p. 90; **Imagestate** p. 34, p. 35 (t); **Mandarin Oriental, Hyde Park, London** p. 19, p. 22; **Oriental Spa, Mandarin Oriental, Bangkok, Thailand** p. 14, p. 18; **Retna/Jenny Acheson** p. 26, p. 33 (t), p. 35 (b), p. 42, p. 43 (b), p. 62; **Retna/Philippe Poulet/Oredia** p. 108; **Retna/Kampfner** p. 100, p. 114; **Retna/Phillip Reeson** p. 45, p. 64, p. 73; **Spa Village, Pangkor Laut Resort, Malaysia** p. 6, p. 12, p. 20, p. 21, p. 61.

Front Jacket: Spa Village, Pangkor Laut Resort, Malaysia.